Disaster Rules

The royalties of this book are donated to Help for Heroes

Disaster Rules

Lieutenant Colonel Rob Russell
MB BS MRCP(UK) FCEM DipIMCRCSEd RAMC
Clinical Lead (Emergency and Critical Care) and Consultant in Emergency
Medicine, Peterborough, and Stamford Hospitals NHS Foundation Trust;
Senior Lecturer in Military Emergency Medicine, Royal Centre for Defence
Medicine; Honorary Senior Lecturer in Emergency Medicine, University of
Birmingham.

Colonel Timothy J Hodgetts CBE QHP
MMEd MBA CMgr FRCP FRCSEd FCEM FIMCRCSEd FIHM
FCMI FRGS L/RAMC
Defence Professor of Emergency Medicine, College of Emergency Medicine;
Honorary Professor of Emergency Medicine, University of Birmingham;
Consultant in Emergency Medicine, University Hospitals Birmingham NHS
Foundation Trust.

Colonel Peter F Mahoney OBE TD
MSc FRCA L/RAMC
Defence Professor of Anaesthesia and Critical Care, Royal College of
Anaesthetists; Consultant in Anaesthesia and Critical Care, University
Hospitals Birmingham NHS Foundation Trust.

Nicholas Castle MSc DipIMCRCSEd RGN SRPara
Nurse Consultant Emergency Care, Frimley Park Hospital NHS Foundation
Trust; Honorary Research Fellow, Durban University of Technology, Republic
of South Africa

Contributors
Surgeon Commander Steve Bland
BSc MB ChB DipMedTox FCEM ROYAL NAVY
Consultant in Emergency Medicine, Queen Alexandra Hospital, Portsmouth;
Medical Director, Defence CBRN Centre, Winterbourne Gunner.

Surgeon Captain Geraint W Evans FRCSEd FCEM ROYAL NAVY
Director of Clinical Studies, Royal Centre for Defence Medicine.

Andrew Thurgood MSc, DipIMCRCSEd DipHS RGN SR Para
Honorary Senior Lecturer, Department of General Practice & Primary Health
Care, Royal Centre for Defence Medicine.

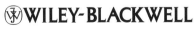
WILEY-BLACKWELL
A John Wiley & Sons, Ltd., Publication

BMJ|Books

Library of Congress Cataloging-in-Publication Data
Disaster rules / Rob Russell . . . [et al.] ; contributors, Steve Bland . . . [et al.].
    p. ; cm.
    Includes bibliographical references and index.
    ISBN 978-1-4051-9378-8 (pbk. : alk. paper)
    1. Disaster medicine–Rules.   2. Emergency management–Rules.   I. Russell, Rob.
    [DNLM: 1. Disaster Planning.   2. Emergency Medical Services.   3. Mass Casualty Incidents.
WA 295]
    RA645.9.D57   2011
    363.34'8-dc22
                                                                            2010036367

ISBN: 9781405193788

A catalogue record for this book is available from the British Library.

This book is published in the following electronic formats: ePDF 9781444329698; Wiley Online Library 9781444329681; ePub 9781444329704

Set in 9.25/12 pt Meridien by Aptara® Inc., New Delhi, India
Printed and bound in Malaysia by Vivar Printing Sdn Bhd

1   2011

Contents

Introduction

This book distils evidence and experience of complex incidents involving multiple casualties into a simple framework, with 'rules' that can be applied to assist in incident management. The rules are generalisations and their exceptions are explained. The term 'major incident' has a different meaning to each emergency service. In health service terms, the definition that this book follows is 'Any incident where the number, severity or type of live casualty, or by its location, requires extraordinary resources' [1].

A major incident can be man-made or natural, simple or compound (interrupts lines of communication and/or transportation; degrades the health service response through infrastructure damage to hospitals and/or ambulances) and compensated or uncompensated. When the resources at the scene remain inadequate to cope with the volume or complexity of the casualties, then the incident is uncompensated – this is synonymous with the meaning of the word *disaster* adopted within this book.

One of the most extreme examples of a modern *disaster* occurred in the aftermath of the earthquake in Haiti on 12 January 2010. Not only were there in excess of 200 000 killed and 300 000 injured, but factors conspired to compound the response to the incident – government buildings were damaged; the local United Nations infrastructure was destroyed; hospitals were part of the incident; and both the principal airport and the port were affected, which restricted the effectiveness of the international aid agency response. The destruction of an estimated 50% of the capital's buildings generated tens of thousands of displaced persons requiring the basic essentials of fresh water, food, sanitation and shelter.

Major incidents are reported, internationally, on a near daily basis; yet, within the UK they are relatively rare (it has been estimated that on average 3–4 multiple casualty situations occur per year, with a range 0–11 [2]). Therefore, local experience is likely to be limited. These easy-to-remember rules may unfreeze the inertia that is inevitable when faced with an overwhelming crisis and help the individual to order their thoughts.

The structure of this book reflects the paradigm developed within the *Major Incident Medical Management and Support* (MIMMS) programme since 1994. MIMMS is a generic, all-hazard training approach to major incidents that has been adopted internationally by civilian emergency services and by NATO: it follows the CSCATTT paradigm (Command-Safety-CommunicationsAssessment-Triage-Treatment-Transport).

The rules in this book are equally applicable when viewed through an alternative lens, the most distributed being the DISASTER paradigm developed in the US following the 9/11 disaster in 2001 (Detect-Incident command-Scene security and Safety-Assess hazards-Support-Triage and Treatment-Evacuation-Recovery) [3]. The section on special incidents is particularly relevant to this CBRN-focused approach.

Whatever paradigm you follow, rules are only a guide. The ability to be flexible and adaptable during a major incident remains essential. Nevertheless, rules provide you with a reference point from which to start, a benchmark and confidence from which to improvise in the most challenging of circumstances.

R Russell
T Hodgetts
P Mahoney
N Castle
2011

References

1. Advanced Life Support Group. *Major Incident Medical Management and Support: The Practical Approach*. London, BMJ Publishing; 2002, 2nd edition.
2. Carley S, Mackway-Jones K, Donnan S. Major incidents in Britain over the past 28-years: the case for the centralised reporting of major incidents. *Journal of Epidemiology and Community Health* 1998; **52**: 392–398.
3. National Disaster Life Support Foundation. Accessible at: www.ndlsf.org.

CHAPTER 1

Golden Rules

!	Rule 1:	Every incident is different, but the solutions are the same
!	Rule 2:	Prior planning and preparation prevents poor performance
!	Rule 3:	When exercising, start small and build up
!	Rule 4:	No plan ever survives first contact with the enemy
!	Rule 5:	Disasters do not respect borders: cross-border agreements must be in place
!	Rule 6:	Children can get hurt too

Rule 1: Every incident is different, but the solutions are the same

The potential variety of major incidents is huge. Consider the immediate environment in which you work: how many potential sources of a major incident are there? Now expand this area geographically to include the local region/county/state and then the country in which you work: how many other sources did you consider?

Even at high-risk locations, such as a chemical factory or airfield, it is unrealistic to predict exactly where an incident will occur, and what the environmental conditions will be like when it happens (e.g. day or night, weather, wind direction). It is neither plausible nor desirable to write a plan with the detail to cover all eventualities. Even if you could produce such a plan, it would be unreasonable to expect all relevant stakeholders to read it all – let alone remember the detail and apply it in a crisis.

As a result, major incident response plans should be 'all-hazard' and based on a common structure of priorities. If the same priorities are applied consistently, then plans will be constructed in a similar way, personnel will find them easier to navigate, experience will be analysed and deconstructed with a common logic, and learning (individual and organisational) is likely to be reproducible. A response, when necessary, will be standardised and follow best practice.

This is the same principle adopted for resuscitation of the seriously ill or injured patient: <C>ABC [1].

The following hierarchy of priorities can be used in any circumstance that generates multiple casualties [2]:

Command and control
Safety
Communication
Assessment
Triage
Treatment
Transport

CSCATTT is the <C>ABC of major incident management. These principles can be used at the scene or at a hospital, and in a military or civilian environment. The principles provide a systematic response to any incident, natural or man-made, irrespective of its type.

If you remember nothing else, remember CSCATTT.

References

1. Hodgetts TJ, Mahoney PF, Russell MQ, Byers M. ABC to <C>ABC: redefining the military trauma paradigm. *Emergency Medicine Journal* 2006; **23**: 745–746.
2. Advanced Life Support Group. *Major Incident Medical Management and Support.* London, BMJ Publishing; 2002, 2nd edition.

Rule 2: Prior planning and preparation prevents poor performance

Or *'Better to prevent and prepare than repent and repair'*

Or *'To fail to plan is to plan to fail'*

This time-honoured military saying is self-explanatory: anticipation of the likely challenges posed by any task, before they arise, enables sensible planning for how those challenges can be met. The attitude 'It will never happen to us' is no defence for poor planning.

The importance of thorough and effective planning is demonstrated by the actions of Major General Sir Frederick Roberts during the Second Afghan War.

MILITARY EXAMPLE
The Second Afghan War

The Second Afghan War (1878–1881) had gone badly for British Forces, culminating in disaster at Maiwand on 27 July 1880: the Berkshire Regiment lost their colours, and were almost wiped out, as were two regiments of loyal Sikh Cavalry. The British garrison at Kandahar immediately came under siege. The main British force at Kabul seemed powerless to help them. Roberts volunteered to lead 10 000 troops to relieve Kandahar, 313 miles away, in the heat of the Afghan summer.

Roberts had already demonstrated the value of meticulous preparation the previous year. Hugely outnumbered by Afghan fanatical holy warriors (Ghazis) at Sherpur, but aware that the Ghazis liked to attack under cover of darkness, he took the precaution of laying in large supplies of star-shells, newly developed at the Royal Ordnance Factories. He set up his riflemen on a ridge overlooking an open plain, and kept them at high readiness. As 100 000 Ghazis launched their 'surprise' assault across the plain, they were lit up by the star-shells, making easy targets for the rifles. Roberts' victory was total.

Tasked with relieving Kandahar, he planned his march with equal thoroughness. He formed a 'Transport Corps' to manage water and food supplies on the march, and to convey heavy equipment over the mountainous terrain. So successful was his organisation that Roberts brought his force to Kandahar in 22 days, intact and in fighting order. They engaged and defeated the besieging Afghan army on 1st September.

The variety of possible major incidents demands an 'all-hazard' approach with maximum flexibility (Rule 1); however, this should not be misinterpreted as vague planning. An acute receiving hospital will have a common core plan (the 'all-hazard' response), but may also have a series of supplements containing detail for specific high-risk incidents within the area of the hospital's responsibility – for example, an incident generating large numbers of children, large numbers of burns, or casualties that have been exposed to toxic chemicals or radiation.

Specific high-risk sites (airport; chemical installation) will demand their own plan for a major incident. A mass gathering is a frequent and predictable risk for multiple casualties, and national guidance exists for those preparing the medical response plans at sports stadia and music events [1, 2]. Common principles of major incident management can still be followed to structure these plans (Rule 1).

Consider the high-risk sites or events in your area that could produce a major incident. Does each location have a plan that is regularly rehearsed and reviewed? Is there consistency between the plans in their structure and scope of content? Does each plan conform to published national guidance or statute (such as the Civil Contingencies Act 2004 [3])?

References

1. Department for Culture Media and Sport. *Guide to Safety at Sports Grounds*. London, HMSO; 2008, 5th edition. Accessible at: www.culture.gov. uk/images/publications/GuidetoSafetyatSportsGrounds.pdf.
2. Health and Safety Executive. *Event Safety Guide: A Guide to Health, Safety and Welfare at Music and Similar Events*. Norwich, HSE Books; 1999.
3. Civil Contingencies Act 2004. Accessible at: http://www.cabinetoffice. gov.uk/ukresilience/preparedness/ccact.aspx.

Rule 3: When exercising, start small and build up

When designing a major incident exercise, it is tempting to plan for what is perceived to be the most realistic scenario: a multi-agency exercise with simulated casualties. This approach, like a man building his house on sand [1], does not first secure the foundations of education (Figures 1.1 and 1.2): it runs the risk of not testing the plan but the staff, who will feel under personal pressure. Without an understanding of the fundamental principles of a major incident, response staff may resent and disengage from the exercise, thus reducing or negating its value.

Most front-line personnel, outside the major incident planning core team, will have a limited working knowledge of the procedures involved within a major incident. The cognitive understanding and psychomotor skills that front-line staff need should be taught or refreshed prior to a multi-agency exercise.

Knowledge and understanding can be built through lectures or an online training programme; practical skills (such as triage or the use of a radio) can be acquired individually; decision-making and judgement can be assessed through a tabletop exercise. This stepwise approach to learning allows staff to have built their competencies in a controlled environment and to participate with confidence in a multi-agency exercise with simulated casualties (when there is little or no opportunity to interrupt the flow of activity for structured education). Staff will also be empowered to give more informed feedback on how the plan worked.

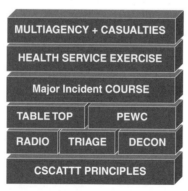

Figure 1.1 The structured approach to major incident exercises. PEWC, practical exercise without casualties.

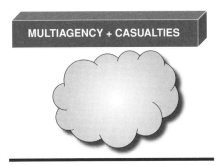

MULTIAGENCY + CASUALTIES

Figure 1.2 The unstructured approach to major incident exercises.

The merit of advertising a multi-agency major incident exercise is debatable. Advertising the exercise, and potentially offering the required training in the interim, removes personal and corporate anxiety, and allows adequate preparation. This preparation builds confidence in roles and procedures and moves the focus away from individual performance to the performance of the plan and the collective response. However, experience has demonstrated that those off-duty may not be contactable when the planned exercise occurs, particularly when this is out of normal working hours.

Not providing warning of exercise would seem to be a better test of the response as a genuine incident will arise without any advance notification. However, rumour usually leaks out, regardless of precautions to the contrary, and this can cause broad apprehension of staff. Should they check the plan and their roles? Of course they should, but false rumours degrade morale and those in key roles will feel under personal pressure: again, this may threaten disengagement and reduction in the effectiveness of the exercise.

Rule 4: No plan ever survives first contact with the enemy

Viscount Slim of Burma

Although planning is essential (Rule 2), plans must be flexible enough to be adapted as the situation changes. Rigid adherence to plans that have been made irrelevant by events can have disastrous consequences.

An example of inflexible planning is provided from the fall of Singapore, 15 February 1942.

MILITARY EXAMPLE

The Fall of Singapore

Plans for defending the vital British Naval base in Singapore were almost entirely designed to meet an attack from the south. A northern assault across the straits from the Malayan mainland seemed impossible as Malaya was in British hands. The plans also assumed British naval superiority. The loss of HM Ships Prince of Wales and Repulse to air attack and the dramatic speed of the Japanese occupation of Malaya left the 'impregnable fortress' of Singapore vulnerable to attack from the north. Japanese forces crossed the straits and despite valiant resistance conquered the island in just 7 days.

Therefore, to be optimally effective, major incident plans must be as follows:
- Flexible and able to allow for deviation from an expected course of incident evolution, encouraging real-time decision-making
- Easy to follow during an incident
- Inclusive of local knowledge
- Adjusted to learn lessons from previous exercises and incidents
- Subject to annual review
- Based on individual, role-specific action cards

A major incident plan acts as the framework for an organised response. Pitfalls in planning are as follows:
- A plan that relies on individuals: the presumption is that they never take leave or are unwell. Each role should have a number of people prepared to take it on.

- A plan that ignores the possibility of clinical areas being unavailable.
- An activation procedure that does not empower 'front-line' personnel to declare a major incident.

Within the emergency services and at hospitals, the on-call system allows senior managers and clinicians to have major incident roles that are flexible and are allocated at the time of the incident.

The exceptions to this include the roles adopted at a mass gathering major incident, which are predetermined and both staff and equipment may be pre-positioned. The potential pitfall in this circumstance is that whilst the advanced determination of roles allows for a prompt and comprehensive response (by individuals nominated for roles in command, triage and treatment), it is possible that key personnel may already be casualties and be unable to fulfil their role. Therefore, shadow appointments should be made for mission critical roles.

Rule 5: Disasters do not respect borders: cross-border agreements must be in place

A major incident may cross health district, county, state or national boundaries: consider particularly a natural disaster (e.g. earthquake, flood) that will not respect these artificial boundaries.

By definition, a major incident demands extraordinary medical and rescue resources. These will be drafted in from other local emergency services, or even other countries. Examples of international collaboration are: the resources from England supporting the crash site of Pan Am Flight 103 in Lockerbie, Scotland (1988); the existing plans for mutual support between England and France for rail incidents that occur in the Channel Tunnel; and the dual response of French and Italian resources in the Mont Blanc tunnel fire (1999: the separate management of the two halves of the tunnel by independent French and Italian companies is a major factor cited in the failure to provide a concerted response).

Where cross-border cooperation occurs, the predictable complexity of managing a major incident will likely be compounded by differences in language, precedence of emergency services (for example, some countries in Europe have the Police as the lead agency, while others have the Fire Service), triage systems, medical equipment and drugs, treatment protocols, and the scope of practice of pre-hospital care providers (for example, France has a physician-based system; the UK has a paramedic-based system). Therefore, any opportunity for international joint planning and training is likely to be beneficial: remember that 'no time in preparation is wasted'.

Local working

Effective scene control demands that at the scene of an incident where different ambulance services and medical teams are working together, an individual takes the lead. Command of the respective emergency services is effected through 'Incident Commanders' (Silver Commanders) and their deputies ('Forward Incident Commanders', or Bronze Commanders).

Silver and Bronze Commanders should be sufficiently experienced decision-makers: however, all staff should respect the post, irrespective of the post-holder's rank or normal appointment.

Problems can occur where the chain of command is unclear or medical personnel refuse to follow instructions. At the Kegworth air crash on the embankment of the M1 Motorway (1989; 49 dead, 74 injured), there were ambulance resources from more than one service, an unclear health service command structure, and duplication of the casualty clearing station function [1, 2].

International working

The activation of medical resources to assist a distant country is a humanitarian act and there are frequent examples following, in particular, devastating, uncompensated natural disasters such as earthquakes and tsunami (see definitions in *Introduction*). The more common cross-border working relationships between adjacent countries are less visible, but they are no less important.

Differences in national laws in an international setting are a potential for friction:

(a) *Example: Drug therapy.* Internationally, the UK is one of the few countries that allows diamorphine (heroin) to be used for the treatment of pain. A UK medical team carrying diamorphine would need to be cognisant of not breaking the laws of the country they are supporting.

(b) *Example: Medical interventions by non-doctors.* Internationally, training of nurses and paramedics differs and this is reflected in procedures that they are allowed to undertake (even under medical supervision). The potential for disaster within the Channel Tunnel has required a special understanding to be created regarding intervention by UK ambulance paramedics, as French law restricts invasive procedures to doctors only.

Equipment

Across national and state/county boundaries, ambulance services predictably operate different vehicles with different equipment scales, stored in a non-standardised manner. Lack of interoperability of equipment is likely; manifest most simply as different heights and widths of ambulance stretcher that cause difficulty in securing the stretcher when placed in an alternative ambulance.

References

1. Malone W. Lessons to be learned from the major disaster following the civil airliner crash at Kegworth in January 1989. *Injury* 1990; **21**: 49–52.
2. Casualty rethink after rail crash disaster. [Editorial] *Emergency Nurse* 2001; **9**:4.

Rule 6: Children can get hurt too

Ambulance services and emergency departments are used to dealing with sick and injured children, but rarely more than one or
two critical cases at any given time. Evidence from major incidents
shows that children are consistently involved [1–4] and some incidents predominantly involve children (Table 1.1).

Most major incident exercises, both pre-hospital and at hospital,
do not involve children as mock casualties because of complications
over regulations and their welfare during the exercise. If children
are involved at all during incident play, then dummies are likely to
be used, reducing the element of realism.

These factors may mean that neither the emergency system nor
its personnel are fully prepared for the impact that a significant
number of children will have on them. Dealing with children generally engenders more anxiety among rescuers than dealing with
adults. This will predictably result in over-triage, which may be
compounded by any failure to understand the physiological differences between young children and adults (see Rule 33) – specifically, over-triage will occur if personnel are only familiar with adult
triage systems. While over-triage may serve in rapidly evacuating

Table 1.1 Major incidents predominantly involving children

Year	Location	Incident	Deaths
1966	Aberfan, Wales	Slag heap collapse engulfs Pantglas Junior School	144 (116 children)
1996	Dunblane, Scotland	Dunblane Primary School shooting incident	16 children + 1 teacher
1999	Colorado, USA	Columbine High School shooting	12 children + 1 teacher
2002	San Giuliano di Puglia, Italy	Earthquake involving school	26 children + 1 teacher
2004	Beslan, North Ossettia	Militants take 1100 hostages (777 children) in Beslan school	Estimated 396, including 186 children

children from the scene, it will dilute the limited resources available at most hospitals that should be focused on the genuinely needy.

Therefore, both hospitals and ambulance services need to have a paediatric element to their plans: this must include a scale of equipment. At the scene, casualty distribution must take into account the suitability of local receiving hospitals when determining the destination of critically injured children. Paediatric Intensive Care is not universally available. Those hospitals without a Paediatric Intensive Care Unit (PICU) must consider how this capability may be rapidly improvised on a temporary basis, pending transfer to a PICU at a time when ambulance resources are stretched.

Following natural disasters or a refugee crisis, a significant proportion of patients requiring medical treatment will be children and many of these children will require feeding and treatment for infectious illnesses [5]. This should be taken into account in any response planning.

References

1. Wardrope J, Ryan F, Clark G, Venables G, Crosby C, Redgrave P. The Hillsborough tragedy. *BMJ* 1991; **303**: 1381–1385.
2. . Brown M, Marshall S. The Enniskillen bomb: a disaster plan. *BMJ* 1988; **297**: 1113–1116.
3. Hodgetts T, Hall J, Maconochie I, Smart C. Paediatric triage tape. *Pre-Hospital Immediate Care* 1998; **2**: 155–160.
4. Hines K, Hines W. The Aberfan disaster: 21 October 1966. *Pre-Hospital Immediate Care* 2000; **4**: 53.
5. Parke T, Haddock G, Steedman D, Pollock A, Little K. Response to the Kurdish crisis by the Edinburgh MEDIC 1 team. *BMJ* 1992; **304**: 695–697.

CHAPTER 2
Command and Control Rules

! Rule 7:	Convert chaos to mild confusion	
! Rule 8:	Good morale results from conscientious leadership	
! Rule 9:	Even when all appears lost, keep your nerve and keep going	
! Rule 10:	A major incident for one emergency service is not automatically one for the other services	
! Rule 11:	The end of the incident does not end the need for medical support	
! Rule 12:	Disasters are dynamic – it is already happening	
! Rule 13:	Avoid the massed blue (or red) disco lights	
! Rule 14:	There are few bad decisions worse than indecision	

Disaster Rules 1st edition. © Rob Russell, Timothy Hodgetts, Peter Mahoney and Nicholas Castle. Published 2011 by Blackwell Publishing Ltd.

Rule 7: Convert chaos to mild confusion

The scene of a major incident will initially be one of chaos. The aim of the Incident Commanders should be to manipulate this situation to one with some semblance of order as rapidly as possible. Complete order is unachievable, at least until the last patient has left for hospital and the role of the health services at the site scales down.

This requirement for organisation is the reason for 'Command and Control' taking precedence in the hierarchy of priorities (see Rule 1). Without the framework of command and control, the efficiency of the response will not be optimal, no matter how well other individual priorities are managed.

Command works vertically within each emergency service. Chains of command must be established and adhered to. The Police, Fire and Ambulance Services have clearly defined rank structures. As more senior officers arrive at the scene they will take over command of their respective service.

This clear structure does not exist amongst doctors. The absolute seniority of the Medical Commander is much less important than the training and experience (s)he has to perform this function. The first doctor at the scene will become the acting Medical Commander. This role should change hands as little as possible as, with each handover, vital information may be lost. Ideally, there should be only a single handover, medical command passing to the doctor who has been pre-determined to attend the scene in this role. In many regions in the UK, there is now an established pool of doctors with the requisite training and experience.

The doctor replaced as Medical Commander should ideally be allocated a task nearby as they remain a source of potentially vital situational awareness.

Control operates horizontally across the services. The Police have overall control of the Silver area and are the lead agency in UK. In other countries (e.g. Sweden, The Netherlands), the Fire Service takes overall control. This difference is unimportant: what is important is that all personnel understand and respect the individual national policy.

As long as the Bronze area is considered unsafe, the Fire Service will invariably maintain control within the area until the danger has been neutralised. Either the Fire Service or Police may control the cordon surrounding this area of hazard (the 'inner cordon') to account for all emergency service personnel entering and leaving the area.

Rule 8: Good morale results from conscientious leadership

> Yet trained in camps, he knew the art,
> To win the soldier's hardy heart.

Marlowe

MILITARY EXAMPLE

The last fight of General Sir Ralph Abercromby Alexandria, 21 March 1801

This battle by the British Army of the Nile against Napoleon's forces was very nearly lost – and would have been, but for the extraordinary tenacity of the British troops.

At one point the 28th (Gloster) Regiment were fighting French infantry in front, while repelling cavalry behind. In the heat of battle, Abercromby was mortally wounded, and briefly unconscious. His first words on coming round were to insist that the blanket he was using as a pillow should be returned to the common soldier who had given it to him. He then refused to be taken from the field for treatment until victory was secured, fearing the effect that his removal might have on his men's morale.

Abercromby died of his wounds seven days later. His obituary in the London Gazette stated: 'By his steadfast concern for the welfare of those under his command, he inspired ordinary men to deeds of extraordinary courage'.

It was Abercromby's victory on land through exemplary leadership, combined with Nelson's victories at sea, which ensured the failure of Napoleon's campaign in the Middle East.

From the military perspective, good morale will stem from a belief in what you are doing, a belief that others value what you are doing (colleagues and seniors; the public), confidence in your leaders, confidence in your equipment, and confidence in your immediate mutual support (whether this is fire support from your buddies, or reliable medical treatment if you are injured). The analogies for those working in the hostile environment of a major incident are clear.

An effective manager gets things done:an effective leader inspires others to get things done.

An investment in team morale is possible within the preparation cycle for a Major Incident and will pay dividends in the crisis. Opportunities to meet, work and train with other potential commanders and team members are not only opportunities to rehearse roles, but opportunities to build team competence, cohesiveness and confidence – thereby building morale through building relationships. Good leadership requires knowledge of your staff's strengths and weaknesses and an ability to exploit individual strengths.

Rule 9: Even when all appears lost, keep your nerve and keep going

MILITARY EXAMPLES
The 57th Foot ('The Die-Hards') Albuhera, 16 May 1811

This was another near disaster for the British Army, which was averted by courage and resilience. The 57th Foot (later the Middlesex Regiment) kept fighting, despite losing all their Officers and all but seven of their men, killed or wounded. As their Colonel fell, he shouted 'Die hard, 57th, die hard!' from which the Regiment gained its nickname.

The Buffs (3rd of Foot) were in an even worse situation, with only three men left standing at the end of the battle. The Military Historian General Sir William Napier, who had witnessed the battle as a young subaltern, wrote of it many years later, 'Then was seen with what a strength and majesty the British soldier fights'. But perhaps a greater, if somewhat veiled, compliment was paid by the French commander, Marshal Soult, writing to Napoleon: 'I always knew the English were bad soldiers, and now I am sure of it. I had them outnumbered, out-manoeuvred, and out-gunned, but they were too stupid to realise this, and would not run. Eventually, my losses were so heavy that I was forced to withdraw'.

British Field Hospital under Quarantine Afghanistan, May 2002

In May 2002, a small, tented British field hospital was co-located with around 300 British troops on Bagram airbase, Afghanistan. Over the course of 3 days clinical staff were stricken by meningitis (5 cases) and/or severe gastroenteritis (31 cases): two patients required ventilation on intensive care. Five of eight intensive care nurses and the only intensive care consultant were affected. Surgery was suspended and the two surgeons worked as general physicians; the sole emergency physician (author TH) was additionally required to be the responsible consultant for intensive care treatment and ward treatment (there was no general physician, given the small size of the unit) – his personal log on Day 3 records 'Feel like Lt Chard at Rourke's Drift'.

The British camp (hospital and co-located personnel) was quarantined. An inner quarantine was established, separating out staff from the tent where the sickest patients were clustered. Drugs ran acutely low and resupply was provided from allied American, French and German military facilities in the area. Clinical personnel were drafted in as an emergency from the British field hospital in Oman. The medical crew who evacuated the first ventilated casualty to the UK became symptomatic and personnel were admitted to an infectious disease unit. The working diagnosis was verocytotoxic E. coli: after 10 days the diagnosis was confirmed as a new strain of norovirus, with no previous record of the virus behaving in this way.

Very often, the successful resolution of a crisis depends not on knowledge, or even experience, but on the strength of will and character to keep working even when the odds against success seem impossible. Whilst knowledge and skill are essential to the success of the health service response to a disaster, the ability to persevere and do 'the most for the most' when faced with overwhelming numbers of injured and scarce resources is just as vital.

Linked with this, flexibility and resourcefulness are valuable attributes for commanders especially when, despite careful training and preparation, the incident is not evolving in line with planned contingencies (Rule 4).

Rule 10: A major incident for one emergency service is not automatically one for the other services

The Health Services definition of a major incident is one in which the live casualties by their number, severity, type or location require extraordinary resources [1].

Incidents that produce a large number of dead and few live casualties may have only a limited impact on medical resources, but will involve a large Police and possibly Fire Service response. The air crash over Lockerbie (1988) is an example of this type of incident, with Police required to secure a very large area of crash site and Fire Service required to manage the fires and casualty rescue in Lockerbie village [2–3].

Can large numbers of dead impact acutely on the health services?

Those that die at the scene are the responsibility of the Police, with a procedure to remove the deceased from the scene directly to a designated 'temporary mortuary' for forensic examination (e.g. an aircraft hangar with associated sanitation, radiography and body-cooling capability).

Hospital services are therefore theoretically unaffected by managing the dead from a major incident. In practice, this is not always the case.

Following the Buj earthquake (2001) in Gujarat, India, the public transported large numbers of bodies to the nearest hospital in Ahmedabad for declaration of death (>20 000 killed; 167 000 injured).

On a smaller scale, the British field hospital in Helmand Province, Afghanistan, was receiving the coalition military dead (including Afghan National Army and Afghan National Police) from the Province in the intense sustained conflict during the summer of 2009: the capacity of the mortuary was reached and a rapid contingency was required to be developed. This model uses hospital staff to receive, examine, certify and care for the dead prior to repatriation, with a heavy associated psychological burden over an extended period.

The Dunblane Primary School shooting (1996) was a significant incident for both the Police and Health Services, but did not require an extraordinary response from the Fire Service.

At an individual hospital level there is a predictable requirement for a 'media major incident'. This may be the result of a local health scare that generates substantial media interest, demands a public helpline to be rapidly established and manned, and requires management action to effectively contain and inform the media that respond to the hospital – but this does not affect normal clinical service delivery.

Any major incident (with or without casualties) will likely generate an initial response from all three main Services. Where an individual Service is not needed it will rapidly scale down. As the Police have the duty of investigation, their presence is likely to be enduring after the hazard control and casualty rescue phases (see Rule 11).

References

1. Advanced Life Support Group. *Major Incident Medical Management and Support: The Practical Approach*. London, BMJ Books; 2002, 2nd edition.
2. Steedman D, Gordon M, Cusack S, White M, Robertson C, Little K. Lessons for mobile medical teams following the Lockerbie and Guthrie Street disasters. *Injury* 1991; **22**: 215–218.
3. Redmond A. The work of the south manchester accident rescue team (SMART). *Injury* 1990; **21**: 21–24.

Rule 11: The end of the incident does not end the need for medical support

In the initial phase of a major incident, there is an escalating response from all the emergency services with the aim of saving and preserving life. Even after all live casualties have been removed from the scene there will be a requirement to maintain a level of medical support, while other services continue forensic investigation, then site clearance.

Examples of incidents that have demanded an extended commitment from the emergency services are the body recovery work at 'ground zero' following the Twin Towers terrorist incident in New York, 11 September 2001; and natural disasters such as major earthquakes (Buj, India, 2001, 167 000 killed; Muzaffarabad, Kashmir, 2005, 79 000 killed) and the Indian Ocean Tsunami (2004; estimated 230 000 killed).

On-scene response

The removal of the last live casualty from the scene signals a reduction in medical cover required. However, medical support is still required during the incident recovery phase to deal with any injuries sustained by the emergency services, to pronounce death with further bodies that are recovered, and in the event an unexpected live casualty is discovered. Following the Moorgate underground train crash (1975), it was 12 hours before the last survivor was freed and five days before the body of the driver was recovered [1].

In natural disasters the focus shifts from emergency life-saving intervention in the first 48 hours to public health and prevention of disease (provision of clean water, sanitation, shelter, food and immunisation) in the enduring incident-recovery phase.

In-hospital response

The emergency department (ED) is the common point of entry to the hospital where there is triage to identify the most needy for intervention in the ED, for imaging, and for definitive care (surgery and/or intensive care).

The impact on a hospital is unlikely to be short-lived and may affect the ability to sustain the same level of routine services [2]. Patients may require multiple returns to the operating theatre for repeat debridement, particularly those that have suffered heavily contaminated wounds after an explosion. A high level of surgical activity was sustained for five days across the acute receiving hospitals in Thailand following the Asian Tsunami: here, wounds were also heavily contaminated and wound infections were common in hospitals that ignored principles of war surgery and undertook primary closure [3].

Regional and national resources can also be stretched, with implications for coping with casualties from normal daily background activity. Following the Ramstein Air Show disaster (1988), around 500 people required hospital treatment, many with burns: the number of burns patients outstripped the number of burns beds available in Europe. Burns unit and burns intensive care resources are consistently limited: nightclub fires provide a periodic challenge to deal with multiple burns patients (Gothenburg, Sweden, 1998, 63 killed and 200 injured; Buenos Aires, Argentina, 2004, 194 killed and 714 injured; Bangkok, Thailand, 2009, 61 killed and 212 injured).

Enduring support

There will be an increased demand on local and regional rehabilitation services, and hospital outpatient follow-up may be undertaken for years. Psychological consequences may be slow to emerge, but once evident are certainly likely to be slow to resolve. Many individuals see experience of a major incident as a tipping point in their lives, with 'life before' and 'life after' the event.

Rowles *et al.* demonstrated that following the Kegworth air crash (1988) 10% of patients were seriously disabled or in a persistent vegetative state at 12 months [2].

References

1. Hines K, Hines W. Moorgate underground disaster: 28th February 1975. *Pre-Hospital Immediate Care* 2000; **4**: 79.
2. Rowles J, Learmouth D, Tait G, Macey A. Survivors of the M1 air-crash: outcome of injuries after 1 year. *Injury* 1991; **22**: 362–364.
3. Lennquist S, Hodgetts T. Evaluation of the response of the Swedish healthcare system to the tsunami disaster in South East Asia. *European Journal of Trauma and Emergency Surgery* 2008; **34**: 465–485.

Rule 12: Disasters are dynamic – it is already happening

A major incident is not a static event: problems and challenges will evolve and emerge over time.

Emergency service resources will also evolve: personnel and tasks will need to be redistributed and reallocated. Command roles will change. Snap decisions will be made, but flexibility needs to be retained to allow a change in a chosen course of action.

There is a balance between flexibility to change and repeated ineffective decision making: the military adage 'Order, counter-order, disorder' identifies how conflicting instructions will lead to a breakdown in confidence of the chain of command and a loss of discipline.

The first personnel on scene must demonstrate leadership and establish the framework of command and control that supports the process for analysing problems and challenges systematically and gives a structure for prioritising what will initially be limited resources. The framework for decision-making is the 'CSCA' paradigm (Rule 1). For the Health Services this means avoiding being drawn into direct patient contact: Triage, Treatment and Transport must wait until other resources are available.

There are two clear exceptions to this rule. The first is a context where other resources will be delayed or unavailable, when it will be necessary to progress through the CSCATTT paradigm: an example is the military combat setting where, for tactical reasons, care on the ground is provided by the embedded personnel without need for reinforcement (other than for evacuation). The second is where resources are already in place before the incident – this is the specific advantage of preparing to respond at a mass gathering event. A range of capabilities are used at mass gatherings from first aid responders from the Voluntary Aid Societies (e.g., St John Ambulance Service) [1] through to comprehensive, physician-led on-site resuscitation facilities [2–3].

Where medical treatment facilities and/or equipment dumps are pre-designated at a mass gathering, it is possible that these may be damaged or destroyed by the incident: contingency plans for secondary locations are required.

References

1. Cheshire N, Gill D. An analysis of the activity of a crowd doctor at a premiership football stadium. *Pre-Hospital Immediate Care* 1998; **2**: 199–200.
2. Chesser T, Norton S, Nolan J, Baskett P. What are the requirements for medical cover at motor racing circuits. *Injury* 1999; **30**: 293–298.
3. Russell R, Hodgetts T, Castle N. Medical support to an organised rave. *Pre-Hospital Immediate Care* 1999; **3**: 10.

Rule 13: Avoid the massed blue (or red) disco lights

A sea of blue (or red) flashing lights is a common televised image of massed emergency service vehicles at a major incident – yet, this is directly in contrast to what is desired to happen [1].

Standing operating procedures call for all emergency vehicles, with the exception of designated control vehicles, to turn off their engines (fire appliance engines will remain switched on to power their pumps), turn off their flashing lights and leave their keys in the ignition [2].

The rationale for this directive is to be able to clearly identify command vehicles, the rallying point for each service and the incident commanders. The first ambulance, fire and police units at the scene will act as the initial incident command vehicles, until the designated and specifically designed and equipped vehicles arrive for each service (in some areas there is agreement for services to share the same vehicle). Depending on the incident site, the initial vehicles may continue to act as a Bronze Command point thereafter.

Tabards (vests) identifying service commanders will often not be immediately available: the flashing vehicle lights will help commanders locate each other and facilitate the development of a combined emergency command structure.

Keys are left in the ignition so that vehicles can be moved quickly if necessary and so that specific drivers do not have to be found and summoned from their other duties.

Failure to follow this rule increases the risk of confusion and will impact adversely on effective command and control at the scene of the incident (highlighted at the Kegworth air crash in 1989 [1]).

References

1. Malone W. Lessons to be learned from the major disaster following the civil airliner crash at Kegworth in January 1989. *Injury* 1990; **21**: 49–52.
2. Advanced Life Support Group. *Major Incident Medical Management and Support: The Practical Approach*. London, BMJ Books; 2002, 2nd edition.

Rule 14: There are few bad decisions worse than indecision

Major Incident Commanders for each of the emergency services will make many decisions during a major incident. These decisions are based on the best available information and situational awareness at any given point in time. This is the concept of 'bounded rationality' where decisions are made on incomplete information, but it is judged to be enough information.

Events during a major incident are time-critical: a delay in decision-making because of a desire for further confirmatory evidence must not be allowed to paralyse the command and control process. Indecisiveness within the command chain will result in personnel doing 'their own thing', which is not likely to represent the best use of resources.

Potential commanders at all levels may develop the speed and accuracy of decision-making by regular practice during realistic training exercises. Whilst full-scale exercises are important, they are time consuming and expensive to coordinate. There is much value in using a tabletop model or a command exercise on the ground without casualty play: both of these encourage synthesis and analysis of information to develop judgement and decision-making. They also allow time to be contracted or expanded, where this improves the training value.

Tactical advisors can provide immediate advice to senior officers in Gold and Silver positions to improve the quality of information on which decisions are made. In addition, working with appropriate specialists from outside the emergency services such as rail transport companies, the port authority or airport management (at rail, harbour and airport incidents, respectively) provides location-specific advice as well as expert incident knowledge: however, incident command remains with the 'blue light services'.

Commanders are accountable for the decisions they make. Even with the best intention and preparation, not every decision will be proven to be correct. It is easy to criticise in retrospect, but many decisions will be made on incomplete information and an evolving situation. Good documentation provides protection and justification for the decisions made (remember: 'Good notes, good defence; poor notes, poor defence; no notes, no defence!').

Contemporaneous notes can be regarded as evidence and it can be expected that notes, logs, diagrams and photographs will be required to be presented for a police investigation. Coroner's Inquests and Public Inquiries may not occur until months or years after an event when memories are selective and predictably incomplete: your contemporaneous notes will be invaluable should you be called as a witness – or, more worryingly, as a defendant.

CHAPTER 3
Safety Rules

! Rule 15:	Follow the *1-2-3 of Safety*	
! Rule 16:	A place of safety may be a false haven	
! Rule 17:	Mother Nature produces the mother of all disasters	
! Rule 18:	Rescuers will become casualties	

Disaster Rules 1st edition. © Rob Russell, Timothy Hodgetts, Peter Mahoney and Nicholas Castle. Published 2011 by Blackwell Publishing Ltd.

Rule 15: Follow the *1-2-3 of safety*

Whether attending the scene in the immediate aftermath or as part of the matured response to an incident, all rescue workers will face danger. If rescuers are to perform their roles safely, all existing and potential hazards must be identified and neutralised, or at least managed within acceptable boundaries of risk.

The *1-2-3 of Safety* is a hierarchy of priorities:

1 **Self**. Am I safe?
2 **Scene**. Is the scene safe? Are those approaching the incident protected from becoming part of the incident?
3 **Survivors**. Have both the injured survivors and uninjured survivors been removed from further danger?

Personal safety must come first, especially for healthcare workers. Health workers are a valuable resource: becoming a casualty will demand further treatment resources to be tasked, will adversely affect staff morale, and will fail to provide (and delay) the initial intended patient care.

Where risks need to be taken to rescue casualties it is more appropriate that those with the training, equipment and experience to manage hazards undertake this – in most systems this is the Fire Service. An exception is the military combat setting: here there is absolute reliance on the courage of individual soldiers to rescue their colleague or buddy from a gun battle, minefield or burning vehicle. Contemporary history has frequently recorded such selfless acts.

Personal Protective Equipment (PPE) provides a basis for protection: if personnel deploy to the scene without the correct PPE their access should be prohibited through the outer cordon. This is more likely to be seen with individual medical staff responding to offer assistance: statutory emergency services should have the requisite PPE. At any large incident a proportion of those involved will be off-duty healthcare personnel: these professionals will invariably demonstrate leadership and initiative to help the injured in the early aftermath, but for their own safety they should be relieved by appropriately equipped personnel as soon as is practical.

In the recommendations following the Clapham rail disaster (London, 1988; 35 killed, 500 injured) it was stated that all emergency services must provide effective PPE [1]. After the Cannon Street rail incident (London, 1991; 2 killed, 524 injured) the lack of standardisation of healthcare services' clothing was again identified [2].

Despite these formal recommendations, McGregor *et al.* identified in 1997 that 21% of hospital-based mobile medical teams did not provide eye protection and 22% did not have access to protective trousers [3]. Although 94% of mobile medical teams did have access to protective footwear, this was typically of a low protective standard (rubber Wellington boots with no reinforced toe cap). This historical poor level of preparation in the UK (extending from equipment through training and pre-hospital experience) is an underpinning reason to have moved away from reliance on *ad hoc* hospital-based teams to maintaining a local pool of trained, experienced, equipped pre-hospital care practitioners (specifically, doctors affiliated to and accredited by the British Association for Immediate Care).

A further necessity is situational awareness of the hazards in the environment: safety is an essential part of the commander's briefing to staff as they report on scene for duty.

References

1. Hidden A. *Investigation into the Clapham Junction Railway Accident.* London, HMSO; 1989.
2. New B. Too many cooks? *The Response of the Health-Related Services to Major Incidents in London.* London, The Kings Fund Institute; 1990, Research Paper No 15.
3. McGregor P Driscoll P, Sammy I, Kent A, Maloba M, Nancarrow J. Are UK mobile medical teams safe? *Pre-Hospital Immediate Care* 1997; **1**: 183–186.

Rule 16: A place of safety may be a false haven

Hospitals are understandably regarded as a place of safety for the injured, but a natural disaster will not discriminate between a hospital and any other building. Where a hospital is part of the incident, then the incident can be regarded as 'compound'. The implications are that the effectiveness of the local response is undermined and the complexity of the external assistance required is increased – international guidelines recommend a field hospital must be in place within 24 hours of an incident if it is to make an impact on survival from acute trauma, where the window of opportunity is the first 48 hours [1].

Research following the 1971 San Fernando earthquake identified that the majority of deaths occurred due to collapsing hospitals, and the Geological Survey have estimated that up to a third of casualties following a major earthquake in San Francisco would be due to hospital building collapsing [2]. In the devastating earthquakes in Bhuj (India, 2001), Kashmir (2005) and Haiti (2010) hospitals were severely affected, being damaged or destroyed.

Attempts to 'earthquake proof' buildings are limited by cost: effectiveness is also dependent on the severity of the earthquake. Kerr noted that there was a fault with regards earthquake protection design of many American hospitals [3] – and many hospitals in developing countries have none of this protection [4].

This has led to the promotion of the concept of a flexible community-based medical response to provide the initial medical care following a substantial earthquake. Such a response is important when we consider the impact of earthquakes on road and public transport infrastructure that will delay medical/rescue staff reporting to duty as well as hindering patient transfer to hospitals.

An additional benefit of a more flexible community-based response is that it can help to reduce the workload of those surviving hospitals, which may be exceptionally challenged.

However, contemporary history shows that earthquakes have often occurred in the poorest parts of the world where a socially advanced community-based self-help response would seem unrealistic. The earthquake in Haiti (2010), one of the poorest countries on the planet, demonstrated a loss of social structure with a breakdown of police function, and lawless armed gangs on the streets.

There are exceptions, where earthquakes threaten advanced societies, that a community-based model may be more relevant (Japan

– Kobe earthquake, 1995, >6400 deaths; USA – San Francisco earthquakes of 1906 and 1989, >3700 deaths in 1989).

References

1. WHO-PAHO Guidelines for the Use of Foreign Field Hospitals in the Aftermath of Sudden-Impact Disasters. Pan-American Health Organization; 2003.
2. Schultz C, Koenig K, Noji E. A medical disaster response to reduce immediate mortality after and earthquake. *The New England Journal of Medicine* 1996; **334**: 438–444.
3. Kerr R. Bigger jolts are on the way for southern California. *Science* 1995; **267**: 176–177.
4. Guy P, Ineson N, Bailie R, Grimwood A. Op Nightingale: the role of BMH Dharan following the 1988 Nepal earthquake, some observations on third world earthquake disaster relief mission. *Journal of the Royal Army Medical Corps* 1990; **136**: 7–18.

Rule 17: Mother Nature produces the mother of all disasters

'Natural' incidents are different from 'man-made' incidents. They are typically much larger in scale, both geographically and in the resulting number of casualties. In addition, natural incidents are more likely to be *compound*, with a disruption in lines of communication (land lines; mobile telecommunications), lines of transportation (roads, rail and airheads disrupted) and health infrastructure (hospitals and medical centres). All of these factors will delay and/or inhibit the rescue effort and contribute to a protracted incident. In the earthquake in Haiti (2010), both United Nations and national government buildings were destroyed: this greatly undermined the country's ability to coordinate the early response to the disaster.

As it is impossible to control the causative factors associated with natural incidents (floods, hurricanes, earthquakes, volcanoes, tsunami) the destructive power will continue unabated until they have run their course: attempts at rescue will be unsafe if not impossible in this phase.

A natural disaster may generate overwhelming casualty numbers: the incident will be *uncompensated*, with inadequate resources available to treat all casualties optimally. International medical aid may be requested by the affected nation's government to compensate, although the type of aid and where it is deployed must be carefully assessed.

Experience from the Asian Tsunami (2004) that affected Phuket Province in Thailand was that public hospitals close to the affected areas (Khao Lak; Phi Phi Island) wanted and needed assistance, but the needs assessment was confined to the private hospitals of the Province's capital who denied the requirement – the Swedish Tsunami Commission concluded that care was delayed to Swedish nationals in Thailand because of a slow and incomplete response, stemming from an inadequate assessment [1]. There were around 25 000 Swedish nationals in Thailand at the time of the tsunami: 550 were killed and 1500 were injured.

World Health Organisation and Pan-American Health Organisation guidelines identify the first 48 hours as the window of opportunity for treating acute trauma care [2]. However, data from Thai hospitals showed that the surgical response was sustained for at least five days – this is evidence that planning assumptions for external field hospital assistance, or support from overseas medical teams embedded in local healthcare facilities, can afford to be more flexible [1].

Rarely, man-made incidents may be on a scale that overwhelms even the resources of an advanced healthcare system: an example is the Twin Towers terrorist incident on 11 September 2001 (New York; >2900 killed, >6000 injured). Incidents that specifically affect the healthcare infrastructure can also be regarded as examples of a *compound* incident [3].

References

1. Lennquist S, Hodgetts T. Evaluation of the response of the Swedish healthcare system to the Tsunami disaster in South East Asia. *European Journal of Trauma and Emergency Surgery* 2008; **34**: 465–485.
2. WHO-PAHO Guidelines for the Use of Foreign Field Hospitals in the Aftermath of Sudden-Impact Disasters. Pan-American Health Organization; 2003.
3. Hodgetts T. Lessons from the Musgrave Park Hospital bombing. *Injury* 1993; **24**: 219–221.

Rule 18: Rescuers will become casualties

The role of a rescuer is dangerous and inevitably some rescuers will sustain injury [1–3]. It is the responsibility of the emergency services leaders at the scene, the Incident Commanders, to balance the risks to the rescuers with the risks to the incident victims.

During prolonged incidents, when rescuers are working for sustained periods, the need for dedicated support to the rescuers should be anticipated. This is likely during the response to a natural disaster. Gallanter *et al.* (2002) reported that in the response to protracted forest fires, 10% to 20% of firefighters required medical attention on a daily basis: at times this increased to 25% [3] – however, the majority of these had minor injuries and only 0.2% required referral to hospital.

Following the sarin gas attack in the Tokyo subway when members of the Aum Shinrikyo cult released organophosphate in five coordinated attacks (1995; 12 killed, >1000 injured, mostly with temporary visual disturbance), a significant number of rescuers were affected and required hospital treatment [4]. This was in part due to inadequate availability of personal protective equipment.

Predictably, rescuers will also be killed in the line of duty (examples include 9–11 [5], the King's Cross fire [6] and the Oklahoma bombing [7]). Commanders must be alert to the affect on morale of the rescuers: it may be appropriate to remove and replace a complete team (e.g. hospital medical team; fire appliance crew) where a member has been killed, if resources allow this luxury.

In the aftermath of the incident it is imperative that supervisors are alert to the psychological health needs of their staff. There will be a transition in some from 'normal' short-term negative feelings of anxiety and/or guilt to a clinical syndrome of post-traumatic stress disorder (PTSD). Parallels can be drawn with the high proportion of PTSD seen in combat troops who have been exposed to sustained psychological insult (similar in many respects to a major incident, witnessing horrific death and injury including close comrades) [8].

References

1. Schwartz R. Occupational injuries in emergency medical technicians. *Emergency Care Quarterly* 1990; **5**: 29–39.
2. Cone D, McNamara R. Injuries to emergency medicine residents on EMS rotations. *Prehospital Emergency Care* 1998; **2**: 123–126.

3. Gallanter T, Bozeman W. Firefighter illness and injuries at a major fire disaster. *Prehospital Emergency Care* 2002; **6**: 22–26.
4. Baker DJ. The immediate care of casualties following the release of toxic chemicals. *Resuscitation* 1999; **42**: 101–102.
5. Prezant D, Weiden M, Banauch G, McGuinness G, Rom W, Aldrich T, Kelly K. Cough and bronchial responsiveness in firefighters at the World Trade Center site. *The New England Journal of Medicine* 2002; **346**: 806–815.
6. Fennell D. *Investigation into the King's Cross Underground Fire*. London, HMSO; 1988.
7. Hogan D, Waeckerie J, Dire D, Lillibridge S. Emergency department impact of the Oklahoma city terrorist bombing. *Annals of Emergency Medicine* 1999; **34**: 160–167.
8. US Department of Veterans Affairs, National Center for PTSD. Accessible at: http://www.ptsd.va.gov/index.asp.

CHAPTER 4
Communication Rules

! Rule 19:	Failure to communicate is a common failing at major incidents	
! Rule 20:	Communication must be clear, simple and unequivocal	
! Rule 21:	If you hear a whistle, start running	
! Rule 22:	The media is like a small baby: it needs feeding little, but often	
! Rule 23:	The media has its uses . . . and some of them are good	
! Rule 24:	Follow the ABC of media interviews	

Disaster Rules 1st edition. © Rob Russell, Timothy Hodgetts, Peter Mahoney and Nicholas Castle. Published 2011 by Blackwell Publishing Ltd.

Rule 19: Failure to communicate is a common failing at major incidents

Effective command and control requires good communication – *horizontally* between chains of command (i.e. liaison between the emergency services and supporting agencies) and *vertically* within chains of command.

Formal inquiries into major incidents consistently criticise poor communication as a common failing. This is not surprising given the initial complexity and confusion of an incident. The same lessons will often be re-learned.

Communication errors can be categorised as a failure to pass information, a failure to confirm information, or a failure to coordinate information.

An example of failure to pass information was demonstrated at the Bradford football stadium fire (1985; 56 dead, >265 injured). The receiving hospital was only made aware that a major incident was in progress when critically ill patients started arriving [1]. Similarly, following the King's Cross Fire in 1987, the judge leading the inquiry commented, 'I was left with the clear impression that opportunities to pass vital information between the emergency services were missed' [2]; the same theme recurred following the 7/7 bombings in London (7 July 2005; 56 dead, about 700 injured) [3]. If those on the ground do not share information (e.g., the requirement for equipment, drugs or personnel resources), then commanders cannot react to it.

Critical information needs to be confirmed. When someone gives you a number over the phone you will be used to reading this back. On a radio, ask the operator to 'say back' a grid reference, or other important figure (number of casualties; number of dressings to be resupplied). The radio operator may have limited medical training: use the NATO phonetic alphabet to spell out key words ('ketamine, I spell kilo-echo-tango-alpha-mike-india-november-echo').

Information can be expected to spread quickly from the point of an incident in an uncoordinated manner. Members of the public involved in or witnessing the incident will phone, text or twitter almost immediately and this may bypass the emergency services. Following the Paddington rail crash (London, 1999; 31 killed, >520 injured), the main receiving hospital (St Mary's Hospital, Paddington) was first alerted by a member of staff involved in the incident.

Emergency services at the scene must coordinate the information flow relevant to their chain of command: messages should be passed through a single point of contact (the emergency services control vehicle) and should be logged. If healthcare personnel use their own private networks to phone for off-site assistance (equipment, personnel) there is likely to be both duplication of effort and capability gaps where no action has been taken – with no record of decisions and no accountability.

A series of communication difficulties occurred during 9/11 [4]. Radios failed and there was no universal radio net, so the emergency services were unable to talk to each other. This led to the establishment of independent command posts remote from each other. A New York Fire Chief in the North Tower stated to the 9/11 Commission:

> People watching on TV certainly had more knowledge of what was happening a hundred floors above us than we did in the lobby . . . Without critical information coming in . . . it's very difficult to make informed, critical decisions.

In relation to the parallel incident at the Pentagon on 9/11, the investigation recorded [4]:

> Almost all aspects of communications were problematic, from initial notification to tactical operations. Cellular telephones were of little value . . . radio channels were initially oversaturated . . . pagers seemed to be the most reliable means of notification when available and used.

At the Omagh bombing, mobile phones and radios failed initially because of the static electricity, and fibre-optic telephone trunk lines had been damaged by the explosion [5].

The nature of an incident may compromise or preclude the use of some methods of communication: radios may not work in road tunnels, underground railways or in deep mine rescue – unless this has been anticipated and contingency made for this, for example the installation of a 'leaky feeder' aerial system. In the report of the 7/7 terrorist bombing of the London underground [3], it was recorded:

> The Metropolitan Police Commissioner regards the inability of the Emergency Services to communicate underground as "a significant problem for London". This not a novel problem. It

has been recognised as a major weakness for the last 18 years, ever since the official inquiry into the King's Cross Fire in 1988 [2]. Since then, there has been a failure by successive governments to take the necessary action to install underground communications for the transport and emergency services.

References

1. Sharpe D, Foo I. Management of burns in a major disaster. *Injury* 1990; **21**: 41–44.
2. Fennell D. *Investigation into the King's Cross Underground Fire.* London, HMSO; 1988.
3. London Assembly. *Report of the 7 July Review Committee.* London, Greater London Authority; June 2006.
4. National Commission on Terrorist Attacks Upon the United States. *The 9/11 Commission Report.* Washington D.C. Available at: http://www. gpoaccess.gov/911/pdf/fullreport.pdf (accessed 1 March 2010).
5. Potter S, Carter G. The Omagh bombing: a medical perspective. *Journal of the Royal Army Medical Corps* 2000; **146**: 18–21.

Rule 20: Communication must be clear, simple and unequivocal

MILITARY EXAMPLE

The Charge of the Light Brigade Balaclava, 25 October 1854

This remains perhaps the most famous blunder in British military history, although by no means the most catastrophic. At the heart of the error was Lord Raglan's ambiguous order that the Light Brigade should advance on 'the guns'. This order was the fourth in a series of confusing messages, issued in quick succession. He apparently meant a small battery on the hillside near the British lines. By the time the order reached Lord Cardigan, commanding the Light Brigade, via three intermediaries, it had transformed into an order to attack the main body of Russian artillery, nearly two miles away in the middle of much larger enemy forces. Despite the suicidal nature of the task, Cardigan obeyed the apparent order without question, and 505 men died. The charge had no impact on the battle whatsoever, other than to boost Russian morale.

In the heat of the moment, human beings may mishear or misunderstand orders or messages. The apocryphal World War I order 'Send reinforcements, we're going to advance' became 'Send three-and-four pence, we're going to a dance' after being passed by word of mouth. In a more contemporary example, attributed to Hines [1], a request for 'Entonox' (a mixture of nitrous oxide and oxygen) passed up the human chain from an underground railway platform to the surface was interpreted as a requirement for an 'empty box'.

The simpler and clearer the message, and the fewer the 'communications nodes' through which it passes, the less likely it is to be misinterpreted. Written messages rather than verbal messages will be less open to misinterpretation.

Remember 'CAB' when composing a message:
- Be **C**oncise.
- Be **A**ccurate.
- Be **B**rief.

This approach, allied with good radio procedure (remembering a steady **R**hythm, controlled **S**peed of speech, adequate **V**olume, and the need to avoid a low **P**itch), will reduce message error.

Effective voice procedure includes the phonetic spelling of important words (Rule 19); reducing error in number interpretation ('thirteen' could be misheard as 'thirty' – so spell out long numbers, 'One hundred and thirteen, figures one-one-three'); and breaking down long messages into sections to confirm each key component is understood by the receiver ('Acknowledge so far, over'; 'Say back grid, over').

In the report into the Clapham rail disaster (London, 1988), delay by the London Ambulance Service in mobilising medical teams from local hospitals (St George's, St Stephen's) was identified, together with confusion and delay at St George's, the principal receiving hospital, regarding the declaration of a major incident. This led to recommendations for standardisation of alert messages passed to hospitals (with a move away from colour-coded alert messages to clear text – i.e., to replace 'Amber alert' with 'Major incident declared, activate plan'), and the requirement for hospitals to regularly exercise their communication procedures for a major incident [2].

References

1. Winch R, Hines K, Booker H, Ferrar J. Report following the Moorgate train crash on 28 February, 1975. *Injury* 1976; **7**: 288–291.
2. Hidden A. *Investigation into the Clapham Junction Railway Accident*. London, HMSO; 1989.

Rule 21: If you hear a whistle, start running

Many forms of communication will prove useful at the scene of a major incident. All have relative advantages and disadvantages.

The whistle is a useful communication tool to draw everyone's attention: the expected response is that people will stop what they are doing and listen for a command. However, continuous blasts on a whistle are a signal within the UK Fire Service to *get out now*.

Radios are the most commonly used method of communication. The major advantage of radios is that a predetermined net is used, which assigns 'call signs' to key appointments, encourages discipline within each single service command structure and facilitates the maintenance of a central log of messages. Radios do require training in voice procedure (Rule 20) and cannot be employed if there is considered to be a risk of a radio-controlled secondary device at a terrorist incident. A specific disadvantage is that only one individual can speak at a given time: there will be considerable competition to use the radio.

Mobile phones are more familiar for most people to use than a radio and will be ubiquitous – few professionals will be without their own phone. This can contribute to a loss of coordination of medical messages if the on-site health services control point is uninformed of decisions made with off-site individuals or agencies.

The cellular telephone system has a finite capacity and this capacity can be expected to be exceeded in large incidents. The emergency services may be unable to communicate effectively because of the high volume of public calls. In this circumstance in the UK, the police may instigate Access Overload Control (ACCOLC), which allows modified mobile phones to operate on restricted cells while denying access to general users.

The London Ambulance Service, present at Aldgate station in the series of bombings on 7 July 2005, asked for ACCOLC to be activated because of serious communication difficulties [1]: this was turned down by the Gold Coordinating Group because of the concern of inducing public panic and uncertainty of whether key ambulance officers on the ground had enabled phones. Despite this, the City of London Police was also suffering severe communication problems and activated ACCOLC within a 1 km area around Aldgate station. The police were later criticised because of the impact on other users: it was estimated that between several hundred thousand and a million attempted public calls were lost [1].

Face-to-face communication is essential for Silver and Bronze Commanders both within and between emergency services. Regular meetings of the Silver Commanders should be held to facilitate joint working; commanders will also need to brief new staff face-to-face and allocate them to tasks accordingly.

The use of runners at the scene and within a hospital is common. Written messages should be handed to the runner (Rule 20) and the runner should understand whether a reply is required or not. Even if a response is not needed, the runner must return to the sender to confirm that the message has been passed.

Hand signals can be effective over medium distances, especially if the environment is noisy. Signals may mean different things to different people – advanced agreement and practice is advisable during the training and preparation phase for a major incident: there will be no opportunity once the incident is underway.

Some incidents offer enhanced opportunities. Sports stadia, railway stations and airports will often have public address systems and message screens that may be used for general announcements and directions to the crowd. A loudhailer (bullhorn) can be an effective tool when used sparingly [2]:

> A battalion fire chief also had a bullhorn and travelled to each of the stairwells and shouted the evacuation order: All FDNY, get the f∗∗∗ out!
>
> North Tower, 9/11 terrorist incident

References

1. London Assembly. *Report of the 7 July Review Committee*. London, Greater London Authority; June 2006.
2. National Commission on Terrorist Attacks Upon the United States. *The 9/11 Commission Report*. Washington D.C. Available at: http://www.gpoaccess.gov/911/pdf/fullreport.pdf (accessed 1 March 2010).

Rule 22: The media is like a small baby: it needs feeding little, but often

The national and international media interest in a major incident is extensive and this attention can be intrusive. Victims of the 7/7 London bombing stated that they would have liked protection from unwanted media intrusion, particularly those who were in hospital and those who were interviewed or photographed during or immediately following the incident [1].

Management of the media requires coordination by trained personnel, a stream of reliable information, the setting of boundaries, and respect for the needs of the media in relation to both deadlines and access to credible sources [2, 3].

While the media is usually respectful of boundaries, if no provision is made for regular briefings from official sources, then they may improvise and stretch acceptable professional etiquette. In the 1995 Oklahoma City bombing, a female journalist wore full operating theatre dress to get through the police cordon and gain access to the triage area [4]; and in the Kegworth air crash in 1989, a journalist used operating theatre dress to gain access to hospital wards [5].

Both Horsfall, after the Bradford fire [2], and Evans, after the Clapham rail crash [3], noted that the initial response of the media to a mass casualty incident was overwhelming and that it impacted on the response. Early control of the media is a managerial priority and should be an integral part of any major incident plan.

Dealing with the media at the scene is a Police responsibility, although the other emergency services will also provide subjects to be interviewed. If any casualty figures are to be released they should be cleared first with the Police, to ensure consistency.

Hospitals will have a Press Officer who is trained and experienced in dealing with the media. A Media Reception Point should be identified and a suitable area for filming that gives the television crew sufficient background activity without intruding on patient privacy. Different media elements have different needs – television needs moving images and a clear line of sight to the incident (a camera positioned on a bridge 500 m from a railway accident can still zoom into the activity); radio relies on the background noise for its atmosphere; and print media want time to interview key personalities (professionals and victims).

When providing information to the media, it is important to be mindful of their deadlines and concerns. In the era of 24-hour news channels, it is desirable to give brief updates regularly, rather than long infrequent conferences. *Feed them little, but often.*
Once it is safe and appropriate for journalists to be allowed onto the scene or into the hospital, it is important to be unbiased in selecting who will be permitted access if necessity demands this must be restricted [1]. A policy is to ask the media crews present to choose from their number: it is expected that this *media pool* will then share the information (photographs; digital video).

References

1. London Assembly *Report of the 7 July Review Committee*. London, Greater London Authority; June 2006.
2. Horsfall B. The Bradford disaster: coping with a media invasion. *Health and Social Service Journal* 1985; **95**: 934.
3. Evans R, Perkins A. In case of emergency...the Clapham rail disaster provided St George's Hospital with a tough test of its major incident plan. *Health Service Journal* 1989; **99**: 948–950.
4. Spengler C. The Oklahoma city bombing: a personal account. *Journal of Child Neurology* 1995; **10**: 392–398.
5. Nocera A, Newton A. Bogus doctor deceptions during multi-casualty events and disasters. *Prehospital and Disaster Medicine* 2000; **15**: 125–126.

Rule 23: The media has its uses . . . and some of them are good

Not all aspects of the media's attention are negative: the media can perform a public service function [1, 2] to alert the public and/or members of the emergency services, and hospital staff, to report for duty.

Following the Hillsborough football stadium disaster (1989), the local media in Sheffield was used to request attendance of doctors to the stadium to provide medical assistance, as well as alerting off-duty hospital staff that they should report for duty [3]. At the Enniskillen bombing (Northern Ireland, 1987; 12 killed, 63 injured), off-duty staff were made aware by the media of the terrorist incident that occurred at the town's war memorial during a Remembrance Day ceremony – this was particularly beneficial as a large number of casualties arrived very quickly at the hospital and the call-in system was struggling to contact staff [4].

Examples of public information are traffic advisory messages across local and national radio stations and, in the event of a chemical leak, information for local residents regarding the need for evacuation or the need to stay inside with shut windows (if an evacuation was needed, the police would be obliged to clear houses door-to-door).

After the Clapham train crash (1988), there was a strongly positive impact of the wide media coverage on volunteer blood donors coming forward, resulting in a surge in supply that was essential to the continuing surgical response [2].

For the media to undertake a public service broadcasting role, it requires media representatives to be involved in major incident planning through regional and national Media Emergency Forums. The value of these forums was apparent on 7 July 2005, when a number of issues that had previously been raised in the London forum were managed effectively as a result (e.g., the plan to establish a Media Centre) [5].

However, senior officials have been skeptical regarding the value of media public service broadcasting. The Metropolitan Police Commissioner has said after the 7/7 London bombings [5]:

> I think we have to be quite careful here. The media are not a public service broadcasting operation. That is not how they work; certainly not in London or anywhere else that I am aware of.

and the Mayor of London echoed these sentiments [5]:

> Although on the day I think the media did absolutely the right thing and got the message out, that is on the day, but that is the only time we are on the same side . . . Only on the day of the tragedy does the Press stand with us; all the rest of the time they are our critics. That is the dynamic tension.

References

1. Horsfall B. The Bradford disaster: coping with a media invasion. *Health and Social Service Journal* 1985; **95**: 934.
2. Evans R, Perkins A. In case of emergency . . . the Clapham rail disaster provided St George's Hospital with a tough test of its major incident plan. *Health Service Journal* 1989; **99**: 948–950.
3. Wardrope J, Ryan F, Clark G, Venables G, Crosby A, Redgrave P. The Hillsborough tragedy. *British Medical Journal* 1991; **303**: 1381–1385.
4. Brown M, Marshall S. The Enniskillen bomb: a disaster plan. *British Medical Journal* 1988; **297**: 1113–1116.
5. London Assembly. *Report of the 7 July Review Committee*. London, Greater London Authority; June 2006.

Rule 24: Follow the ABC of media interviews

Commanders and other senior staff must expect and prepare themselves to give interviews to the media. Wherever possible, formal media training should form part of the preparation for a senior role at a major incident.

When giving an interview, there are ground rules to follow. The cardinal rule is to follow your *ABC of media interviews*:

* **A**nswer the question.
* **B**ridge the gap to what you want to say.
* **C**ommunicate your key messages.

As a professional, you need to *answer the question*; politicians may choose to adopt a different approach, where 'answer the question' is replaced with 'block the question'. However, the question may not be the one you wish to answer, so *bridge the gap* and use your answer as a springboard to *communicate your key messages*.

If possible, take time to ready yourself. Take off blood-soiled gloves and apron, straighten your tie and your hair, reflect on the likely questions and your answers – the public want to see and hear a calm professional who is in control.

A microphone should always be presumed to be live. Avoid making any unguarded 'off the record' comments that you would not be happy to hear on the national news: there is no 'off the record'.

Ask what the first question will be before the interview starts. This will give you a short time to think about your answer, build your confidence for the rest of the interview and give a good first impression. The public will only remember a fraction of what you say: what they will remember is how you say it.

Restrict your answers to those things you have been directly involved in. Do not allow yourself to become engaged in speculation.

CHAPTER 5
Assessment Rules

> **!** Rule 25: One is the same as none for planning purposes
>
> **!** Rule 26: You cannot rely on off-duty staff responding to help
>
> **!** Rule 27: Oxygen is a finite resource – and it is heavy
>
> **!** Rule 28: All major incidents are uncompensated at the beginning

Disaster Rules 1st edition. © Rob Russell, Timothy Hodgetts, Peter Mahoney and Nicholas Castle. Published 2011 by Blackwell Publishing Ltd.

Rule 25: One is the same as none for planning purposes

'One is none' is a contemporary Dutch military aphorism. If you rely on a single piece of equipment in either the pre-hospital or hospital environment, you are highly vulnerable to breakage or malfunction. The more essential the item, the more important it is to have a spare readily available.

This vulnerability is likely to be compounded in the field hospital setting (civilian disaster site or military combat operations) where necessity demands that equipment is held at the minimum scale to balance capability with manoeuvrability.

When there is heavy reliance on technical equipment at the field hospital to optimally manage critical trauma, then any loss of capability (in a trauma system that has a long supply chain into a hostile environment) will have a profound effect on how clinicians can manage patients.

All of the following technical equipment is in use in the British field hospital in Afghanistan from 2009 to provide optimal care in a hostile environment (or 'good medicine in bad places') – direct digital radiography; computerised tomography (CT) scan; ultrasound (for focused abdominal sonography in trauma (FAST) of the abdomen; for line and nerve catheter placement; for diagnostic purposes); thromboelastography to monitor the presence and response to treatment of coagulopathy; laboratory analysers for biochemistry, haematology and blood gases; controlled temperature platelet agitator to sustain fragile platelets; and rapid blood product defrosters to provide timely plasma and cryoprecipitate during frequent massive transfusions of the seriously injured.

Resilience planning must take into account how a capability can be rapidly restored should essential equipment fail – for example, can other field hospitals in the network be mutually supportive; is there a co-located store of contingency equipment to temporarily replace broken or malfunctioning items (military field hospitals will commonly maintain duplicate equipment in a nearby location, should the hospital be damaged or destroyed by enemy action); or is the re-supply chain responsive enough to meet short notice demands?

Electrical items in a field setting require a reliable power source: power, and a *back-up* power supply, is a critical consideration when planning to deliver a hospital capability.

Battery-powered devices are also vulnerable, and radios are a good example. Regular checking and correct maintenance of batteries is essential to ensure maximum battery life when needed. When you are issued with a radio, always ask for a spare battery, and whilst checking the radio, ensure that you know how to change the battery. Some battery types have a 'memory effect': if they are used infrequently and recharged after only partial discharge, the proportion of the battery that stores energy becomes progressively smaller.

A complicating factor at the multiple synchronous terrorist bombs in London, 2005, was the lack of planning by the ambulance service to be able to support concomitant major incidents at more than one site [1]:

> The experience of 7 July showed the London Ambulance Service's lack of capacity to deliver equipment and supplies to the scenes of major incidents at multiple sites. As a result of this, there was a lack of basic equipment, such as stretchers and triage cards, and a lack of essential supplies, such as fluids, at the affected Tube stations and at Tavistock Square.

Reference

1. London Assembly. *Report of the 7 July Review Committee*. London, Greater London Authority; June 2006.

Rule 26: You cannot rely on off-duty staff responding to help

The cornerstone of many major incident responses across the emergency services and within hospitals is the reliance on off-duty personnel to drop what they are doing and report for duty. However, selflessness cannot be guaranteed. Consideration needs to be given during the planning phase how to ensure the best staff response, and how to begin to get additional help quickly.

Media coverage of major incidents may use dramatic pictures of staff hurrying to work to attend casualties [1]: such reports can play a part in alerting staff to the situation (Rule 23), but public service broadcasting is generally not the principal mechanism to alert staff. All major incident plans require a call-in system [2].

At the hospital level, the Switchboard can use a group pager or a group text to alert all staff on duty. Most hospitals will follow a prioritised checklist of key appointments to ensure all those on duty (resident and non-resident) have been informed. Some hospitals have an automated system for individuals to confirm a group notification. Where there is a public address system in a hospital, this can immediately and effectively notify all staff.

Within an individual department or ward, it would be expected that off-duty staff are called in through a cascade. This requires an accurate staff contact list to be maintained by each component of the hospital, and for the lists to be easily accessible at all times. It makes sense to call those staff first who live the nearest to the hospital – this will facilitate early practical help.

Cummings and Cone evaluated the willingness of off-duty staff to respond to the hospital [3]. Staff were found to be more willing to respond following a natural incident such as an earthquake (86%), than following a man-made incident such as a terrorist chemical incident (58%).

The same survey found that 30% of staff would have difficulties with unplanned work at the hospital because of childcare responsibilities, with a further 7% citing difficulty because of responsibilities to look after vulnerable elderly relatives. These restrictions were identified when staff were questioned about their ability and willingness to work on past the end of their shift. A further 33% of staff stated pet care as a reason why they would need to go at the normal time!

Andrus and Bogucki surveyed pre-hospital emergency medical personnel and found that 90% had more than one 'mission-critical' job – for example, a job as both a healthcare provider and a voluntary firefighter. Typically, this was with more than one employer [4]. The implications are clear for only being able to respond in support of one service.

By providing a crèche for the children of staff, a hospital may improve the willingness of off-duty personnel to attend during a major incident.

A further consideration is the ability of staff to actually get to their place of work. In a natural disaster, roads will likely be disrupted; furthermore, an individual's over-riding priority may be to look after his/her family – both factors will affect the willingness and ability to attend work. With an incident local to a hospital, road closures and/or security cordons may prevent staff reaching the hospital: in this circumstance, it is necessary to rely solely on those personnel who were present at the hospital at the time of the incident.

An exception is the military field hospital. The principal *raison d'être* of a field hospital is to respond to bursts of casualties. This requires major incident procedures to be regularly invoked and off-duty staff called in to assist. As all staff live adjacent to the hospital and there is often a camp-wide public address system, it is realistic that all off-duty staff will respond within a matter of minutes.

Caution should be exercised in having all staff attend a hospital, or if it is necessary to consider early when staff can be stood down. The major incident is not over once the initial reception and resuscitation is managed in the emergency department: there will be a heavy impact on in-patient services for days or weeks. Thought needs to be given regarding who will be available to start the next shift in 12 hours time.

References

1. Sharpe D, Foo I. Management of burns in major disasters. *Injury* 1990; **21**: 41–44.
2. Brown M, Marshall S. The Enniskillen bomb: a disaster plan. *BMJ* 1988; **297**: 1113–1116.
3. Cummings B, Cone D. Hospital disaster staffing, will they come? *American Journal of Disaster Medicine* 2006; **1**: 28–36.
4. Andrus P, Bogucki S. Multiply committed providers and surge capacity of nationwide emergency medical services. *Prehospital Emergency Care* 2003; **7**: 178.

Rule 27: Oxygen is a finite resource – and it is heavy

Oxygen is a universal resuscitation drug. Common practice is to administer high flow oxygen at 15 L/minute when treating critically ill or injured patients. In order to conserve resources in a multiple casualty incident, it may be necessary to both triage the use of oxygen (limiting its use only for the most needy patients) and to reduce the flow rate – some supplemental oxygen will be better than no oxygen at all.

In a hospital, oxygen and other piped gases may be taken for granted. Ambulance services and field hospitals will rely on cylindered gases, which are bulky and heavy to transport. A conventional steel 'D'-sized cylinder holds 340 L of oxygen – this is a small cylinder, often used in pre-hospital care, and will only allow delivery at 15 L/minute for 22 minutes (see Table 5.1). Modern Kevlar and carbon-composite cylinders are lighter and store more gas per unit volume at a higher pressure: these are clear advantages.

Oxygen concentrators entrain air and selectively adsorb the nitrogen: they are literally a limitless supply of oxygen and are used effectively in remote military medical facilities (field hospitals, ships, and forward surgical teams). The maximum flow rate available will be considerably less than piped or cylindered gas (maximum around 5 L/minute), and a power source is required.

Multi-patient oxygen hubs are marketed for use in major incident and disaster scenarios. Here, a central oxygen source feeds multiple outlets to patients in a casualty clearing station or other improvised medical treatment facility. The use of a liquid oxygen source delivered in a vehicle trailer allows up to 15 L/minute of oxygen to be delivered to 30 patients concomitantly for 2 hours.

Table 5.1 Cylinder life [1]

Cylinder type	Capacity (L)	4 L/min	8 L/min	10 L/min	15 L/min
C-size	170	42.5 min	21.25 min	17 min	11.3 min
D-size	340	85 min	42.5 min	34 min	22.6 min
E-size	680	170 min	85 min	68 min	45.3 min
F-size	1360	340 min	170 min	136 min	90.6 min
G-size[a]	3400	850 min	425 min	340 min	226.6 min

[a]G-size cylinders are very heavy and are typically used only in-hospital.

Although oxygen is in itself not combustible, it does support combustion and, therefore, should be used with care during confined space rescue – especially if cutting equipment is to be used.

Reference

1. Eaton J. *Essentials of Immediate Medical Care*. Edinburgh, Churchill Livingstone; 1999, 2nd edition.

Rule 28: All major incidents are uncompensated at the beginning

An incident is *uncompensated* when the resources are overwhelmed. Most major incidents will start uncompensated, with the exception of when resources are deliberately positioned for an anticipated threat, such as at a mass gathering. In many cases, particularly in the developed world, adequate resources will be quickly mobilised and the incident will become *compensated*.

Exceptions are the true disasters that occur after natural events (such as an earthquake) – it may be days or weeks before the needs of many begin to be met – and MASCAL in the military operational setting (MASCAL is the NATO abbreviation for *mass casualties*, indicating that the evacuation system is overwhelmed: resources are finite in the combat situation and there may be no opportunity for immediate reinforcements).

Commanders must continually reassess their need for resources. The initial assessment of casualties does not have to be completely accurate, just accurate enough to begin to mobilise people, treatment equipment and vehicles. Estimates of casualty numbers and severity will be refined as more information becomes available at the scene.

This evolving picture is commonly seen in the real-time media reporting of major incidents. If the health service commander does their job effectively and gets the *right people* (balance of paramedics, nurses and doctors) with the *right equipment* (shelter, light, drugs, clinical consumables; together where necessary with food, water, environmental control, sanitation, decontamination), then there is a timely opportunity to transform the incident to a compensated status.

An exception where high-quality information is vital from the outset is contemporary combat operations. Coalition forces will send a structured radio message from the scene (it has nine components and is referred to as a '9-Liner') to request medical retrieval. As forces operate in remote areas with extended timelines, it is essential to dispatch the right clinical *capability* (different helicopters carry teams with variable clinical competencies from a paramedic through to a specialist doctor, with the highest capability able to offer anaesthesia and administration of blood and plasma) with the right *capacity* (different helicopters have different capacity for stretcher and sitting patients).

Resources deploying to the scene need to be channelled as they approach and controlled. An early component of the scene assessment will be the location for an emergency helicopter landing site (EHLS) and the establishment of a vehicle circuit.

The choice of EHLS location must take account of the slope of the ground, surrounding hazards (buildings, trees, power and telephone lines), and both proximity and accessibility to the casualty clearing station (ideally, ambulances should be able to approach close to the EHLS). The EHLS will require to be marked and policed. Civilian helicopters may not have the capability to fly safely at night to an improvised landing site: where it is possible, night-time marking can simply be at the intersection of vehicle crossed headlights [1] or by using a 'buzz saw' (a chemiluminescent light stick on the end of several feet of string, swung in an overhead circle: in tactical settings, an infrared light stick can be used).

Factors to consider when establishing the vehicle circuit are:

* Have any routes to and from the scene been affected by the incident?
* What is the current local traffic situation?
* Can the public be told to avoid certain routes (Rule 23)?
* Can vehicles be diverted to a marshalling area near the scene and then be called forward as required?

At a mass gathering, the access and egress routes will be planned in advance. However, the mass evacuation and wide, unpredictable dispersal of the general public following a 'big bang' incident will likely result in significant local congestion. This will impede additional resources responding to the scene and ambulances trying to leave the scene with casualties (traffic control measures are usually only instigated shortly before the end of the event so as not to affect local traffic during the incident).

If an evacuation from a mass gathering is planned, as was demonstrated following the bomb threat at the 1997 Grand National horse race meeting (60 000 evacuated), then car parks can be 'locked down' and the public prohibited from using their vehicles to evacuate. This allows for a safe, rapid and controlled evacuation, but may generate the parallel problems of crowd disturbance and public transport pressures.

Reference

1. Hodgetts T, Porter C. *Major Incident Management System*. London, BMJ Books; 2002.

CHAPTER 6
Triage Rules

! Rule 29: Physiological triage is more consistent than anatomical triage

! Rule 30: Triage is dynamic – patients can get better, or worse

! Rule 31: Label the dead or they will keep popping up

! Rule 32: When lightening strikes reverse your triage

! Rule 33: Over-triage of children is common: roll out the tape

! Rule 34: Effective triage for mass casualties is a balance of clinical need with available resources

Disaster Rules 1st edition. © Rob Russell, Timothy Hodgetts, Peter Mahoney and Nicholas Castle. Published 2011 by Blackwell Publishing Ltd.

Rule 29: Physiological triage is more consistent than anatomical triage

Triage systems may be anatomical or physiological. Anatomical systems rely on an assessment of the patient's physical injuries; physiological systems relate the patient's vital signs to a pre-determined priority.

A triage system must be rapid, safe (will not exclude any with serious injury) and reproducible, regardless of the experience of the user.

Anatomical systems require examination of the patient to identify relevant injuries. In some instances this is instantaneous, and is simply pattern recognition – for example, the soldier with bilateral lower limb amputations from an improvised explosive device, who has a window of resuscitation and surgical opportunity (priority T1, immediate). In other cases, anatomical triage requires intuition to know where to focus a rapid examination and the key signs to elicit: it is for this reason that senior clinicians are commonly cited as being necessary to perform triage at hospital [1]. However, even experienced clinicians cannot reliably detect internal injuries by external examination alone: specifically, a soft abdomen does not exclude haemoperitoneum (see Trauma Rules – *Examination of the abdomen is less reliable than flipping a coin* [2]).

Anatomical systems are poorly reproducible between individuals with different clinical experience: a first aider will make different assumptions and decisions than a surgeon.

Furthermore, physical examination requires the patient to be exposed. This takes time and may need more personnel to assist. It also exposes the patient to environmental hazards, particularly the cold.

For all these reasons, physiological triage systems may offer an advantage. The vital signs required for physiological systems are rapidly and easily obtained. A reproducible algorithm is then followed, without the figures being open to individual interpretation.

The Triage Sieve (Figure 6.1) [3] is a simple protocol for initial triage that is used at the point of injury. It is taught to professional healthcare workers, but has also been taught to firefighters and individual soldiers [4].

In the purist interpretation of triage, the individual performing the Triage Sieve will not be involved in any treatment. In the military version of the Triage Sieve (Figure 6.1) where scene medical

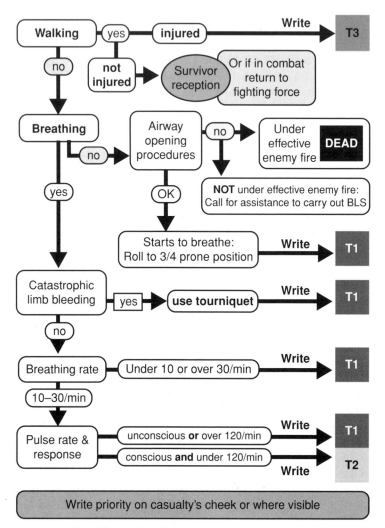

Figure 6.1 The military triage sieve.

resources may remain limited, simple life-saving treatment interventions are undertaken within the Triage Sieve [5].

The Triage Sort [3] is a refinement of the Triage Sieve and takes more time to perform (Figure 6.2). It can be used at the Casualty Clearing Station and on arrival at the hospital, except at times of high patient flow. After the physiological assessment (respiratory

Step 1: calculate the **Glasgow Coma Score (GCS)**

E = Eye opening:	**V = Verbal response:**	**M = Motor response:**
spontaneous 4	orientated 5	obeys commands 6
to voice 3	confused 4	localises 5
to pain 2	inappropriate 3	pain withdraws 4
none 1	incomprehensible 2	pain flexes 3
	no response 1	pain extends 2
		no response 1

$$GCS = E + V + M$$

Step 2: calculate the **Triage Sort score**

X = GCS	**Y = Respiratory rate**	**Z = Systolic BP**
13–15 4	10–29 4	90 or more 4
9–12 3	30 or more 3	76–89 3
6–8 2	6–9 2	50–75 2
4–5 1	1–5 1	1–49 1
3 0	0 0	0 0

$$\text{Triage Sort score} = X + Y + Z$$

Step 3: assign a **triage priority**

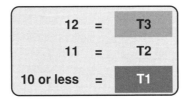

12	=	T3
11	=	T2
10 or less	=	T1

Step 4: Upgrade priority at discretion of senior clinician, dependent on the anatomical injury/working diagnosis

Figure 6.2 The triage sort. (Hodgetts T, Porter C. *Major Incident Management System*. London, BMJ Publishing, 2002.)

rate, blood pressure, Glasgow Coma Scale), the triage officer may upgrade the category if the anatomical findings warrant it – for example, the individual with normal vital signs, but who has been in a fire and has evidence of upper airway burns (may be upgraded from T3 to as high as T1). This is a reason that triage on arrival at hospital should continue to involve senior clinicians, even when physiological systems are used.

References

1. Rosenfeld J, Fitzgerald M, Kossman T, Pearce A, Joseph A, Tan G, Gardner M, Shapira S. Is the Australian hospital system adequately prepared for terrorism? *MJA* 2005; **183**: 567–570.
2. Hodgetts T, Deane S, Gunning K. *Trauma Rules*. London, BMJ Publishing; 1997.
3. Hodgetts T, Porter C. *Major Incident Management System*. London, BMJ Publishing; 2002; .
4. Hodgetts T. *Battlefield Casualty Drills*. Army Code 71638; 2007, 5th edition.
5. Doctrine, Concepts and Developments Centre. *Clinical Guidelines for Operations*. Shrivenham, Joint Defence Publication 4-03.1; 2009.

Rule 30: Triage is dynamic: patients can get better, or worse

Triage is the process by which casualties are allocated a priority. It is a dynamic process and must be repeated at every link of the evacuation chain. Casualties may deteriorate during evacuation or may improve following treatment: the initial category assigned at point of injury may therefore change, and may change more than once.

Triage serves more than one purpose. Initially, it places patients into groups for prioritised treatment at the scene. It will also be used to determine evacuation priorities, which are not necessarily the same as a scene treatment priority – an airway burn may, for example, have no requirement for immediate intervention at the scene, but a high priority for evacuation where elective anaesthesia and intubation is appropriate.

In the contemporary UK military context, triage categories are used routinely even for single patients: this is to ensure the right transport (with the right medical support capability) is directed towards a patient. Additionally, higher risks will be taken to retrieve critically injured soldiers – this is why every soldier is taught the Triage Sieve, in order to consistently identify time critical injury (see Rule 29).

After triage in the ambulance bay, at the hospital (to determine where in the emergency department the patient is to be placed) the concept of prioritising patients continues:

- Triage for order of investigation in the emergency department– there may only be equipment to process one patient at a time (focused abdominal sonography in trauma (FAST) ultrasound of the abdomen; plain imaging of the chest and pelvis).
- Triage for immediate movement to the operating theatre.
- Triage for order in which to go through computerised tomography (CT) scanner.
- Triage for receipt of blood products (if stocks become limited).

Example: Triage is Dynamic

Rail accident. Male casualty, age 35. Chest injury and bilateral fractured femurs.

Bronze Area Triage Sieve:
Not walking, breathing, RR 36, P 128 = **T1**

Initial CCS Triage Sort (for treatment):
RR 40, SBP 80, GCS 12 = **T1**
Treatment: chest drain insertion, bi-lateral traction splints, IV fluids, analgesia.

Second CCS Triage Sort (for transport):
RR20, SBP 100, GCS 15 = **T2**

Rule 31: Label the dead or they will keep popping up

Triage is one of the key priorities in the response to a major incident (see Rule 1). Triage promotes the most efficient use of scarce resources and focuses medical help on those that require it the most.

An essential part of the triage process is applying a label. This indicates to others that triage has been done and the colour codes will direct the treatment teams towards the most needy. The importance of labelling the dead is so that they are neither repeatedly re-triaged, nor are treatment teams diverted to them once death has been declared.

Under normal circumstances, no patient has a higher priority than the patient in cardiac arrest. Non-medical rescue personnel may have a preconceived idea as to how health service personnel will treat patients. This will be particularly true of lay people working as stewards at mass gatherings, who become used to how a static medical team responds to clinical emergencies [2] and who in themselves may have received basic life support training.

Reports from the Hillsborough football stadium crowd crush (1989) highlighted that some casualties received CPR from a second rescuer, after it had already been discontinued. The chaos of this scene was compounded as stewards and police officers performed CPR, as opposed to crowd control.

Dead labels are usually black or white: the date and time of death should be recorded, together with the name of the doctor pronouncing (and the name/number of the police officer witnessing).

The colour codes of triage labels are not universal. This creates the opportunity for misinterpretation when working across boundaries (e.g., across national, State or county boundaries; a civil and military combined response; or where a private organisation interfaces with a statutory service – e.g., a stadium or airport may stockpile different equipment to an ambulance service, if planning has not considered the need for interoperability). Generally accepted UK standards are:

Colour	Descriptor	Priority	Time dependence
RED	Immediate	T1	Cannot wait
YELLOW	Urgent	T2	Can wait
GREEN	Minor	T3	Must wait
BLACK	Dead	Dead	–

A simple mass triage system would be to ask all those that can stand and walk to do so: this identifies the minor (T3) casualties. Of the remainder, those that can raise a limb to command are the urgent (T2). Those that do not respond are the immediate (T1) – or they are dead.

Reference

1. Wassertheil J, Keane G, Fisher N, Leditschke J. Cardiac arrest outcomes at the Melbourne cricket ground and shrine of remembrance using a tiered response strategy: a forerunner to public access defibrillation. *Resuscitation* 2000; **44**: 97–104.

Rule 32: When lightening strikes reverse your triage

It has been estimated that lightening strikes occur at a rate of between 0.09 and 0.12 per 100 000 population per year, with an associated mortality rate of up to one-third [1]. In addition to outdoor mass gatherings, outdoor swimming pools, playing fields and camping sites have all been identified as being high-risk areas for lightening strikes and have the potential to generate multiple casualties [1–2].

In one bizarre incident in Bena Tshadi, Democratic Republic of Congo (1998), all 11 players of one football team were killed instantaneously by a single lightening bolt – 30 other people suffered burns.

Cardiac arrest following lightening strike has a better potential outcome than cardiac arrest due to ischaemic heart disease, even after a prolonged resuscitation attempt [3]. Victims of lightening strike who are still breathing and are haemodynamically stable are unlikely to deteriorate further [1, 4].

At most major incidents, there are few indications for CPR as the chance of a successful outcome is poor – and by diverting resources to unsalvageable patients there is a risk of adversely affecting the outcome of salvageable patients (see Rule 34). However, when faced with multiple casualties following a lightening strike, it is recommended that CPR be started together with appropriate advanced life support (ALS) measures.

References

1. Lederer W, Wiedermann F, Cerchiari E, Baubin M. Electricity-associated injuries II: outdoor management of lightning-induced casualties. *Resuscitation* 2000; **43**: 89–93.
2. Buechner H, Rothbaum J. Lightning stroke injury – a report of multiple casualties resulting from a single lightning bolt. *Military Medicine* 1961; **126**: 755–762.
3. Leibovici D, Shemer J, Shapira S. Electrical injuries: current concepts. *Injury* 1995; **26**: 623–627.
4. Dollinger S. Lightening-strike disaster among children. *British Journal of Medical Psychology* 1985; **58**: 375–383.

Rule 33: Over-triage of children is common: roll out the tape

Triage at the scene of a major incident is designed to maximise the use of resources, to target treatment at the most needy and to ensure timely transfer to an appropriate definitive care facility. The triage of children following major incidents has been criticised as ineffective and experience has demonstrated that receiving hospitals have been overloaded with uninjured children, or children with only minor injuries [1].

The widely available, simple, physiology-based triage tools use the range of adult vital signs to determine triage priorities. Children have vital signs that vary proportionally with their age and length. The smaller the child, the more likely that childhood 'normal' vital signs fall into the adult 'abnormal' range: this will lead to over-triage if adult algorithms are applied to small children.

Specifically, a distressed but uninjured 1-year old child is likely to be triaged as 'T1 immediate' based on the vital signs range of an adult. Perhaps more importantly, a critically ill child will be undiagnosed if clinical staff overcompensate for these differences: in this case, abnormal vital signs may be dismissed as normal variables by the inexperienced, who make incorrect adjustments for a child.

Over-triage can be minimised by using an objective paediatric triage system, such as the Paediatric Triage Tape [2]. This has been validated [3] and uses the child's length as a proxy for age. The tape consists of a linear series of Triage Sieve algorithms with physiological variables that are corrected for the length (and the corresponding age) of the child. The tape is rolled out from the head of the child and is read from where the heel touches the tape (Figure 6.3).

A further factor to consider is the psychological distress that rescuers experience when dealing with injured children, which is also likely to contribute to over-triage. There will be a temptation to clear children quickly from the scene, even if they are not the most seriously injured.

Most receiving hospitals will have limited paediatric capacity. Incorrect triage, and in particular over-triage, may divert limited paediatric resources from those children that need the resources most. Reliable triage of children is therefore not just as important as for adults, it is perhaps more important. This is highlighted in natural disasters and displaced populations when a high proportion of those presenting for treatment are children [4].

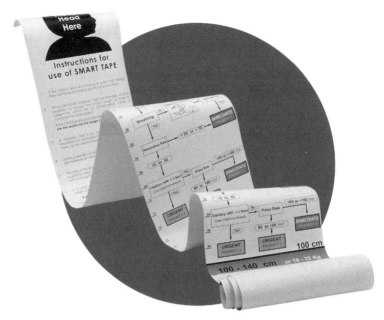

Figure 6.3 The paediatric triage tape.

References

1. Van Amerongen R, Fine J, Tunik M, Young G, Foltin G. The Avianca plane crash: an emergency medical systems response to paediatric survivors of the disaster. *Pediatrics* 1993; **92**: 105–110.
2. Hodgetts T, Hall J, Maconochie I, Smart C. Paediatric triage tape. *Pre-Hospital Immediate Care* 1998; **2**: 155–160.
3. Wallis L, Carley S, Hodgetts T. A procedure-based alternative to the injury severity score for major incident triage of children: results of a Delphi consensus process. *Emergency Medicine Journal* 2006; **23**: 291–295.
4. Parke T, Haddock G, Steedman D, Pollock A, Little K. Response to the Kurdish crisis by the Edinburgh MEDIC 1 team. *BMJ* 1992; **304**: 695–697.

Rule 34: Effective triage for mass casualties is a balance of clinical need with available resources

In most multiple casualty situations, the conventional triage process of categorising patients according to the urgency of treatment can be applied.

In a true disaster (or 'mass casualty') situation, the overwhelming volume of clinical work requires a modification to this approach. The senior surgeon from the Red Cross Hospital in Kabul (Dr Robin Coupland), 1992, recorded how the hospital adapted during a mass casualty event:

Mass Casualties in the Red Cross Hospital Kabul, 1992

I was a team surgeon in one of four teams when we received roughly 600 new casualties over a period of six days. Most were civilians from the vicinity of the hospital. About 250 with small soft tissue wounds were sent home with antibiotic tablets after having received tetanus prophylaxis. They had instructions to return if they developed problems; few did. This was in keeping with a non-operative policy for small soft tissue wounds, but the extreme circumstances did not allow the patients to remain in hospital for observation.

We were able to admit all patients with larger wounds to dress the wound and give fluids intravenously, benzylpenicillin, tetanus prophylaxis and analgesia. Owing to fatigue and the proximity of the battle, we were able to operate only for some hours each day and those with abdominal wounds had priority. The perioperative mortality was high. Those who were rushed into the operating theatre because of the severity of their wounds usually died during or soon after surgery because the admission procedure had become so disrupted that many arrived on the operating table having received insufficient intravenous fluid replacement. After surgery, more died through lack of postoperative supervision.

Much valuable surgical time and energy was wasted. The patients with abdominal wounds who survived were those who required laparotomy for perforation and not for bleeding. The few patients admitted with thoracic wounds whose condition was not stabilised by fluid resuscitation and chest drainage died before they could reach the operating theatre. Most patients with severe wounds of the limbs that required amputation or wound excision had to wait three or four days for their surgery; only those with massive multiple wounds died in the meantime [1].

Reproduced with permission

Based on this experience in Kabul, three lessons were identified for a mass casualty situation:

1 Intravenous fluids and antibiotics buy time for most patients.
2 Patients with severe life-threatening injuries die despite treatment – unless resources (including the number of nursing staff) and the organisation of the hospital infrastructure are adequate.
3 When the hospital infrastructure is disrupted, surgical resources are easily wasted by operating on patients whose prognosis is hopeless – underlining the importance of realistic triage for treatment – and the death rate is unacceptably high among those who should survive [1, 2].

Thus, under extreme conditions, the traditional approach to triage and major surgical intervention can be challenged by an epidemiological approach, where less emphasis is placed on the more spectacular aspects of surgical care that benefit only a few, in favour of some effective care reaching many more with emphasis on adequate first aid and delayed surgery directed at casualties who would die of infective complications if surgery was not performed.

References

1. Coupland RM. Epidemiological approach to surgical management of the casualties of war. *BMJ* 1994; **308**: 1693–1697.
2. Leppaniemi AK. Managing ballistic injury in the NGO environment. In: *Ballistic Trauma*, Mahoney P, Ryan J, Brooks A and Schwab CW (eds). London, Springer; 2005, 2nd edition.

CHAPTER 7
Treatment Rules

> ! Rule 35: You will treat more T3 than T1
>
> ! Rule 36: If staff are of little use to the hospital, they have no merit on MERIT
>
> ! Rule 37: Surgical teams leave with their patients; medical teams stay
>
> ! Rule 38: Medical equipment should be interoperable
>
> ! Rule 39: CPR will rarely be indicated at a major incident
>
> ! Rule 40: Not all patients require surgical intervention
>
> ! Rule 41: Pain is the 5th vital sign: be prepared to treat it
>
> ! Rule 42: After the crush, remember to flush

Disaster Rules 1st edition. © Rob Russell, Timothy Hodgetts, Peter Mahoney and Nicholas Castle. Published 2011 by Blackwell Publishing Ltd.

Rule 35: You will treat more T3 than T1

Major incidents produce casualties with a range of injury severity. For planning purposes, the number of minor injured ('walking wounded') will be far greater than the number of severely injured survivors [1–6].

Consider a terrorist bomb as an illustration. Those close to the point of explosion will be killed or seriously injured, with the principal effects of the blast wave (compression, then re-expansion of air-filled organs), blast wind (traumatic amputation) and thermal pulse (burns) being concentrated over a small area. Fragments from the bomb (these are *primary fragments* and are classified as *pre-formed* if they are packed around the explosive, such as ball-bearings, or *natural* if they arise from the casing of the bomb) will travel over a much wider area and, in a dense crowd, will produce many survivors with injuries. More casualties still, often of a minor nature, will result from glass, wood chippings and stone fragments from the environment (known as *secondary fragments*) that are carried by the blast wind, or from associated falls.

An exception is an aircraft crash, where the majority if not all passengers are killed (see Box).

INFAMOUS AIR CRASHES

- Pan Am Flight 103 mid-air explosion over Lockerbie, Scotland, 1988:

  All passengers and crew killed.

- Air France Flight 4590 tyre burst from debris on Concorde's take-off from Charles de Gaulle airport leading to fuel tank fire and crash, 2000:

  All passengers and crew killed.

- Pan Am and KLM flights collided on the runway at Tenerife airport, 1977:

  583 killed and 61 injured.

In some aircraft incidents, however, there may be considerable numbers of survivors from the related ground incident where the aircraft impacts (Twin Towers and Pentagon terrorist incidents, 11 September 2001; El Al Flight 1862 collision into flats in Bijlmermeer, Amsterdam, 1992).

Medical resources at the scene will necessarily be prioritised to attend to the needs of the most seriously injured. Care of T3 casualties may be reduced to self-aid or buddy-aid, particularly when the incident remains uncompensated. There is less urgency to move T3 casualties from the scene (other than to facilitate early scene control) and there is logic in holding T3 casualties in an area with a component of medical supervision, in the expectation that some may unmask with more serious injuries. These casualties can then be re-triaged and redirected through the evacuation chain – the most dangerous place for them to deteriorate would be while being transported with other T3s (e.g. on a bus, train or flat-bed truck) in the absence of medical support.

In rare circumstances, it would be appropriate to treat T3 before T1. Baron Larrey, who is first attributed with applying the concept of triage, identified amongst Napoleon's injured troops those who could be quickly patched up and sent back to fight: here, the overriding principle was to win the battle. The same attitude would be defensible in contemporary combat zones, for example if a forward operating base (FOB) or platoon house in Afghanistan was under sustained enemy attack – *the best medicine is to win the battle*.

The concept of treating T3 before T1 is known as *reverse triage*. A further analogy is when there is fire aboard a Royal Navy ship. The crew's priority is to tackle the blaze and protect the ship. Medical personnel may again be ordered to treat the minor injured first to quickly release personnel back to duty.

T3 patients may be considered for discharge from the scene. This requires a competent medical examination (e.g. by mobilising local general practitioners to the scene) and appropriate first aid to ensure clinical accountability, together with close liaison with the police to ensure accountability for documentation of witnesses.

As the volume of T3 patients is likely to far exceed the critical cases, and T3 are easier to move (and indeed some will self-evacuate), there is a real concern that those hospitals geographically closest to the incident can lose the capacity to deal with serious cases. This can be prevented by temporarily holding T3 at the scene while determining the most suitable destination hospital: a bus or a train can be used to take T3 out of the immediate area to where there is improved capacity, leaving local hospitals to manage the time-critical patients.

Careful consideration needs to be given to the role of local minor injury units (MIU) and walk-in centres. Whilst these facilities may

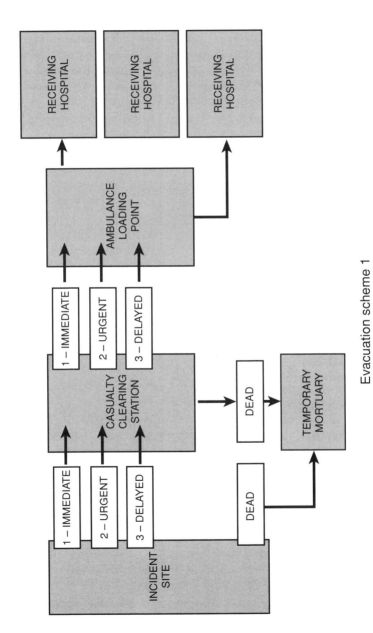

Evacuation scheme 1

Figure 7.1 Casualty flows in compensated and uncompensated incidents.

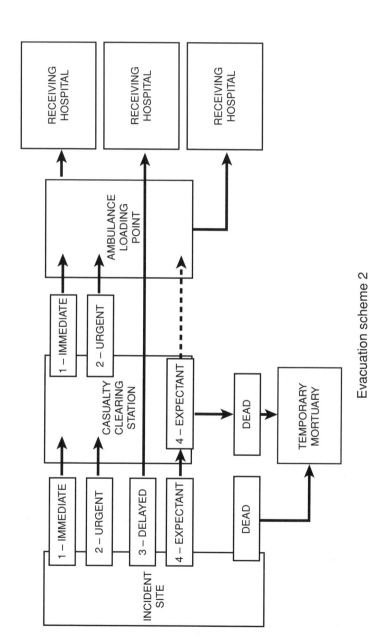

Figure 7.1 (*Continued*)

Evacuation scheme 2

be able to manage T3 casualties, there is no adequate provision for casualties with occult severe injuries, who will reveal themselves over time. Where the mechanism has been severe, undifferentiated minor cases will be best directed to an emergency department with full treatment capabilities (Figure 7.1).

References

1. Allen M. Coping with the early stages of the M1 disaster: at the scene and on arrival at hospital. *BMJ* 1989; **298**: 651–654.
2. Caro D, Irving M. The Old Bailey explosion. *Lancet* 1973; **1**: 1433–1435.
3. Sharpe D, Foo I. Management of burns in major disaster. *Injury* 1990; **21**: 41–44.
4. Stevens K, Partridge R. The Clapham rail disaster. *Injury* 1990; **21**: 37–40.
5. Brown M, Marshall S. The Enniskillen bomb: disaster plan. *BMJ* 1988; **29**: 1113–1116.
6. Lockey D, Purcell-Jones G, Davies C, Clifford R. Injuries sustained during major evacuation of the high-speed catamaran St Malo off Jersey. *Injury* 1997; **28**: 187–190.

Rule 36: If staff are of little use to the hospital, they have no merit on MERIT

It is important that if a hospital has to provide the Medical Commander and/or a Medical Emergency Response Incident Team (MERIT), this does not reduce the ability of the hospital to mount its own response. Ideally, a hospital tasked to provide staff to support the scene should not be the primary receiving hospital – the exception being a field hospital, which may be the only hospital in a single linear chain of evacuation (a field hospital must be more flexible, with the option to project staff forward to support the scene, recover the staff as patients flow to the hospital, and retain additional pre-hospital staff in the emergency department when the scene is clear).

To counter any reduction in capability, there has been a tendency to allocate staff without critical care competencies and/or junior medical staff to MERITs [1, 2]. For example, at one major incident the mobile medical team was made up of a gynaecologist and a communicable diseases nurse [3]. In other examples, hospitals have identified midwifery staff as the key nursing element of mobile medical teams; and emergency departments have been most likely to send their junior nurses as part of a mobile medical team – despite in one documented instance being informed the incident was many miles away from the hospital, so the hospital was not a principal receiving unit [4, 5].

This undermines and undervalues the role of the MERIT. The purpose is not simply to provide extra pairs of hands to duplicate the ambulance service resources, but to enhance the clinical judgement and treatment capability through the provision of the relevant experienced hospital-based specialists.

The requirement is that a MERIT is weighted towards critical care competencies. Those who may be part of a team must have the correct clinical and field training (knowledge of the command and control system; understanding of how to work in the presence of predictable hazards; radio proficiency) and must be familiar with the medical equipment and drugs that they will take with them [2].

An optimal MERIT composition is an emergency physician (team leader skills), an anaesthetist (invasive skills) and two experienced emergency nurses (who are used to dealing with multiple undifferentiated casualties, when diagnoses have yet to be made and treatment pathways are emergent).

If a Medical Commander is required, the medical speciality and seniority of the designated Medical Commander is less important than their possession of specialist training in major incident management and experience at exercises and previous incidents [6].

National Department of Health Guidance on preparing for major incidents has been generic and there is little or no specific guidance on the staffing and equipping (beyond safety equipment) of these teams [7]. This has resulted in wide variations in the equipment carried (see Rule 38) [2, 8].

References

1. Cooke M. Arrangements for on-scene medical care at major incidents. *BMJ* 1992; **305**: 748.
2. McGregor P, Driscoll P, Sammy I, Kent A, Maloba M, Nancarrow J. Are UK mobile medical teams safe? *Pre-Hospital Immediate Care* 1997; **1**: 183–188.
3. Heywood-Jones I. Red alert. *Nursing Times* 1989; **85**: 16–17.
4. Moakes T, Kilner T. Nurses' understanding of their role as part of a mobile medical and nursing team during a major incident. *Pre-hospital Immediate Care* 2001; **5**: 34–37.
5. Coad N, Jones M, Byrne A, Pepperman M. The M1 air crash: the demands placed on anaesthetic and intensive care services of two hospitals. *Anaesthesia* 1989; **44**: 851–854.
6. Simpson A, Laird C. Medical incident officer provision by general practitioners in Scotland. *Pre-Hospital Immediate Care* 2000; **4**: 80–82.
7. Emergency Preparedness Division. *Planning for Major Incidents: NHS Guidance*. London, Department of Health, 2005.
8. Keane C, King G. The varying standards of mobile medical team equipment held by London hospitals. *Emergency Nurse* 2001; **9**: 12–13.

Rule 37: Surgical teams leave with their patients; medical teams stay

The purpose of physician-based teams is to augment the ambulance service competencies by providing refined triage (by overlaying clinical judgment on physiological changes) and advanced resuscitation skills. These teams will be focused at the Casualty Clearing Station (CCS).

The advanced skills are targeted at the management of <C>ABC [1]:

• **C**atastrophic haemorrhage (control of external bleeding using compression dressings and/or topical haemostatic agents [2] and/or tourniquets [3]);

• **A**irway management (including surgical airway and rapid sequence induction of anaesthesia);

• **B**reathing (including intercostal drain, or thoracostomy if the patient is ventilated); and

• **C**irculation (fluid replacement, including blood and plasma).

A physician-based team may be drawn forward from the CCS to an entrapped patient. Requests for a team should be passed through the Forward Medical Commander (FMC) to the Medical Commander (MC): this will ensure control of resources, which otherwise may become dispersed around the scene and fail to be optimally effective.

There are few indications for a surgical team at the scene of a major incident. A surgeon's skills will be of the greatest impact in a functional operating theatre. Most surgical skills that are required for immediate life-saving resuscitation (cricothyroidotomy, intercostal tube drainage, and thoracostomy) are well within the scope of practice of the trained emergency physician or pre-hospital specialist physician.

Where a surgical team may occasionally be required is to undertake field amputation. However, with modern extrication practices and equipment, there is less need than there has been historically. In some circumstances, definitive surgical skills will not be required and the procedure can be adequately performed by the emergency physician and the anaesthetist from a MERIT – for example, should the traumatic amputation be almost complete and release from entrapment achieved by cutting through remaining soft tissue, or if it is simply required to disarticulate a limb of a corpse to gain access to the living.

Should a surgical team be deployed for a specific procedure, the team should accompany their patient back to the hospital to ensure continuity of care. The surgical team should typically comprise a surgeon, anaesthetist and two others, who may be nurses or operating theatre practitioners. The same personal protective equipment and field skills are needed as for the MERIT.

References

1. Hodgetts TJ, Mahoney PF, Russell MQ, Byers M. ABC to <CABC>: redefining the military trauma paradigm. *Emergency Medicine Journal* 2006; **23**: 745–746.
2. Pusateri A, Holcomb J, Kheirabadi B, et al. Making sense of the preclinical literature on advanced hemostatic products. *Journal of Trauma* 2006; **60**: 674–682.
3. Brodie S, Hodgetts TJ, Lambert P, McLeod J, Clasper J, Mahoney P. Tourniquet use in combat trauma: UK military experience. *Journal of the Royal Army Medical Corps* 2007; **153**(4): 310–313.

Rule 38: Medical equipment should be interoperable

And *Equipment levels should build progressively with each enhanced capability*

And *Medical equipment should supplement rather than duplicate ambulance service equipment*

Typically, a single ambulance is equipped to deal with only a small number of casualties as the opportunity to re-supply can be expected after each patient. As a result, its resources will be quickly exhausted in a major incident. This has resulted in ambulance services developing major incident equipment vehicles stocked with consumables (as well as infrastructure support – temporary shelters, signage) to support protracted incidents.

The role of the MERIT is to bring specialist skills to support the ambulance service response and equipment should reflect this, enhancing rather than simply duplicating capability. Having established this, there will be some inevitable overlap of common consumables (airway adjuncts, intravenous cannulae, dressings/topical haemostatics): here, interoperability is highly desirable. An example of best practice is the French system of holding standardised equipment sets for major incidents throughout its national administrative regions: few countries can mirror this across state or county ambulance service boundaries.

A lack of interoperability will be seen during a natural disaster when disparate national and international teams deploy with variable equipment. This hinders integration and flexibility. An exception is the military, where standardisation is a national norm – but interoperability frictions will make cross-boundary working with allies difficult in a crisis, unless there has been opportunity for prior training (important differences include stretcher variants and ambulance/helicopter loading drills; vital signs monitors; drugs; fluids; and documentation).

A medical team's (MERIT) equipment must include the following:

Drugs
- Anaesthetics: local (for nerve blocks) and general
- Analgesics (simple analgesia; opiates, ketamine)

- Fluids (with the option for blood and, ideally, plasma)
- Antibiotics (for open fractures and open abdominal wounds)

Advanced airway management
- Surgical airway
- Adult intubation (including aids to difficult intubation, e.g. disposable optical laryngoscope)
- Paediatric intubation

Ventilation
- Mechanical ventilator
- Chest drain sets (a drainage system using a bag with a one-way valve is more appropriate than an underwater seal in the pre-hospital setting)

Circulation
- Intra-osseous system (limb and sternum access variants)
- Cut down sets (less requirement with intra-osseous availability)
- Central venous access (less requirement with intra-osseous availability: add particular value when undertaking high volume blood product resuscitation, which will be at hospital)

Documentation
- Patient report form (PRF) (alternatives are to use commercial triage tag or ambulance PRF)

POOR DOCUMENTATION IS COMMON

'There was a general failure to maintain records of the response of the emergency services on 7 July. It is understandable that emergency services personnel will be inclined to attend to the urgent and immediate priorities of rescuing the injured, but it is important that records are kept so that lessons can be learnt from the response. It may also be important from the point of view of any investigation or inquiry following a major incident' [1].

All members of the team must be familiar with any equipment that is carried and also with the layout of the equipment within the rucksacks or other mode of carriage. Rucksacks with labelled compartments are generally better than large, heavy boxes: rucksacks are easier to carry, and boxes usually offer less internal equipment organisation (and may have to be emptied to find the desired item).

Reference

1. London Assembly. *Report of the 7 July Review Committee.* London, Greater London Authority; June 2006.

Rule 39: CPR will rarely be indicated at a major incident

The shared primary cause of multiple cardiac arrests at a major incident may be hypovolaemia (penetrating or blunt injuries), traumatic asphyxia (crowd crush) [1, 2], hypoxia (smoke inhalation – Manchester 1985, fire aboard passenger jet, 55 killed; Isle of Man 1973, Summerland leisure centre fire, 50 killed and 80 injured; Gothenburg 1998, discotheque fire, 63 killed and about 200 injured; Perm, Russia, 2009, Lame Horse nightclub fire, >150 killed and about 160 injured), or poisoning (Moscow theatre siege 2002, >170 killed and >700 poisoned by an incapacitating chemical weapon [3]).

The outcome from *traumatic cardiac arrest* has been historically extremely poor [4]. In one US review of 12 462 patients, there were no survivors to hospital discharge. More encouragingly, in a UK 10-year review of 909 patients attended by a helicopter emergency service, the survival to hospital discharge was 7.5%, although patients with hypovolaemia as the primary cause of cardiac arrest had a very poor outcome [5].

No patients who received CPR at the Hillsborough football stadium crush [2], the Oklahoma [6] or Enniskillen bombings [7], or the Clapham train crash [8] survived to hospital discharge, despite a small number of initially successful returns of circulation.

In his inquiry into the Hillsborough stadium incident, Lord Justice Taylor recommended that the minimum medical provision at sports stadia should include the availability of a defibrillator. In most cases, the aetiology of the cardiac arrest at a major incident will be non-ischaemic and the primary cardiac arrest rhythm will be non-shockable. The provision of defibrillators at mass gatherings has, however, saved lives when single victims of cardiac ischaemia have collapsed in the crowd [9, 10].

Whilst most cases of cardiac arrest are non-ischaemic, the sudden collapse of a casualty with minor injuries or a rescuer is more likely to be due to an ischaemic dysrhythmia – and thereby amenable to treatment by prompt defibrillation.

By contrast to civilian experience, contemporary UK military experience has generated a cohort of hypovolaemic cardiac arrest survivors, with a common mechanism being limb loss following improvised explosive device – this outcome is associated with a practice of highly aggressive blood product resuscitation immediately post-arrest.

A specific instance when basic life support is appropriate in the major incident setting is if a patient stops breathing due to iatrogenic administration of opiate analgesia, and ventilatory support is required whilst naloxone is given.

References

1. DeAngeles D, Schurr M, Birnbaum M, Harms B. Traumatic asphyxia following stadium crowd surge: stadium factors affecting outcome. *WMJ* 1998; **97**: 42–45.
2. Wardrope J, Hockey M, Crosby A. The hospital response to the Hillsborough tragedy. *Injury* 1990; **21**: 53–54.
3. Coupland R. Incapacitating chemical weapons: a year after the Moscow theatre siege. *Lancet* 2003; **362**: 1346.
4. Rosemurgy A, Morris M, Olson S, Hurst J, Albrink M. Prehospital traumatic cardiac arrest: the cost of futility. *Journal of Trauma* 1993; **35**: 468–474.
5. Lockey D, Crewdson K, Davies G. Traumatic cardiac arrest: who are the survivors? *Annals of Emergency Medicine* 2009; **48**: 240–244.
6. Hogan D, Waeckerle J, Dire D, Lillibridge S. Emergency department impact of the Oklahoma City terrorist bomb. *Annals of Emergency Medicine* 1999; **34**: 160–167.
7. Brown M, Marshall S. The Enniskillen bomb: a disaster plan. *BMJ* 1988; **207**: 1113–1115.
8. Stevens K, Partridge R. The Clapham rail disaster. *Injury* 1990; **21**: 37–40.
9. Michael JA, Barbera JA. Mass gathering medical care: a twenty-five year review. *Prehospital and Disaster Medicine* 1997; **12**: 305–312.
10. Cooke M, Hodgetts T. The largest mass gathering. *BMJ* 1999; **318**: 957–958.

Rule 40: Not all patients require surgical intervention

The majority of casualties following a major incident will be minor 'walking wounded' (priority T3) who may simply require treatment at the scene or within a hospital's emergency department (see Rule 35). However, survivors from high-energy transport incidents (train crash, plane crash) will predictably have blunt injuries requiring general surgical and/or orthopaedic intervention [1, 2]; and survivors from terrorist bombs will commonly have fragmentation wounds that require debridement.

The Hillsborough stadium crowd crush (1989) resulted in 25 patients with traumatic asphyxia requiring admission to intensive care units for ventilatory support. 159 patients were transferred to hospital from Hillsborough and 66 were discharged from the emergency department after treatment for minor injuries – this means that 28% of in-patient admissions were to intensive care [3]. A disproportionate demand on intensive care beds has also been seen after smoke inhalation (fire aboard passenger aircraft at Manchester airport, 1985) and following mass poisoning with a respiratory depressant (Moscow theatre siege, 2002).

Mass poisoning, demanding a 'medical' rather than a 'surgical' response has also been seen in the civilian context at Bhopal, India (1984, >150 000 required medical care, many with toxic pulmonary oedema, following the accidental release of methyl isocyanate from a chemical factory [4]), and in Tokyo (terrorist organophosphate (Sarin) gas release in the subway [5]).

Experience in the aftermath of a natural disaster is that the emphasis shifts within the first week from the treatment of acute traumatic injuries to the provision of primary care and prevention/treatment of communicable disease. The needs of a population displaced during conflict will also be focused on primary care, and particularly the needs of children and pregnant women.

The UK medical teams supported the Kurdish refugee crisis in 1991. A team from Edinburgh reported that only 44 of 1606 patients treated had traumatic injuries [6]. The team from Manchester described the ubiquitous diarrhoea and scabies; malnutrition in breast-feeding babies; and dehydration in febrile infants. The synergy of emergency medicine and public health medicine is particularly clear in the recovery from these situations [7].

Environmental conditions or infectious diseases may also be responsible for 'medical' major incidents. In 2001, the British Army experienced a major incident due to heat stress amongst troops on exercise in Oman; and in Afghanistan in 2002 an outbreak of Norovirus caused a compound major incident when over 40% of the staff were affected (with symptoms of meningitis and gastroenteritis) closing the UK field hospital on Bagram Airbase.

The psychological aspects of being involved in a major incident cannot be underestimated – many will view their lives in the perspective of life before the incident and life after the incident. Some will be emotionally numbed or hysterical immediately following the incident [8]; many (including rescuers) will develop the symptoms of post-traumatic stress disorder.

Occasionally, rescuers may be so emotionally affected that they have to be relieved of duty. In a report of the Omagh bombing, Northern Ireland (1998) [9], the medical commander noted:

> At one stage a woman was turned over by the Regimental Medical Officer and medic to find a small child lying naked beneath her mother. This caused the emotional collapse of the soldier who was then removed from the scene.

References

1. Stevens K, Partridge R. The Clapham rail disaster. *Injury* 1990; **21**: 37–40.
2. Kirsh G, Learmouth D, Martindale J. Nottingham, Leicester, Derby aircraft accident study group. *BMJ* 1989; **298**: 503–506.
3. Wardrope J, Ryan F, Clark G, Venables G, Crosby A, Redgrave P. The Hillsborough tragedy. *BMJ* 1991; **303**: 1381–1385.
4. Tachakra SS. The Bhopal disaster. *The Journal of the Society of Health* 1987; **107**: 1–5.
5. Okumura T, Takasu N, Ishimatsu S, Miyanoki S, Mitsuhashi A, Kumada K, Tanaka K, Hinohara S. Report on 640 victims of the Tokyo subway Sarin attack. *Annals of Emergency Medicine* 1996; **28**: 129–136.
6. Parke T, Haddock G, Steedman P, Little K. Response to the Kurdish refugee by the Edinburgh MEDIC 1 team. *BMJ* 1992; **304**: 695–697.
7. Redmond A, Jones J. The Kurdish refugee crisis – what have we learned? *Archives of Emergency Medicine* 1993; **10**: 73–78.
8. Collins S. What about us? The psychological implications of dealing with trauma following the Omagh bombing. *Emergency Nurse* 2001; **8**: 9–13.
9. Potter S, Carter G. The Omagh bombing – a medical perspective. *Journal of the Royal* Army Medical Corps 2000; **146**: 18–21.

Rule 41: Pain is the 5th vital sign: be prepared to treat it

The principal vital signs are respiratory rate, pulse rate, blood pressure and temperature – but pain can be regarded as the 5th vital sign [1]. Pain is predictable following injury and the majority of patients, whether their injuries are minor or severe, will require some form of analgesia.

The treatment of pain is a humanitarian intervention that should be regarded as a basic need in a major incident. The severity of pain, and the response to analgesia, can be monitored serially using a pain score. There is a range of scores. Common pain scoring systems are:

- 0–3 (0 = none, 1 = mild, 2 = moderate, 3 = severe)
- Visual analogue scale (mark on a scale from 0 to 100 mm)
- Wong-Baker Faces Scale (drawings of faces from happy to sad)

The smallest significant change when using a visual analogue scale (VAS) is 13 mm [2]; a Faces Scale is particularly useful for children, or those with learning disabilities [3].

The impact of simple, non-pharmacological measures (such as reassurance and splinting) should not be underestimated. The requirement for analgesia following injury can be considered stepwise in accordance with the World Health Organisation's pain ladder, although this tool was designed for use in palliative care:

- *Step 1: Mild pain*. Use non-opioid simple analgesics (e.g. paracetamol, ibuprofen).
- *Step 2: Moderate pain*. Use oral opioid analgesics (e.g. codeine, tramadol).
- *Step 3: Severe pain*. Use opioid analgesics (e.g. fentanyl intravenously or transmucosally; morphine intravenously) and other strong parenteral analgesics (e.g. ketamine intravenously).

Ketamine is a safe, effective, rapid-onset and offset analgesic for use in both pre-hospital care and emergency department settings [4, 5]. Analgesic doses are 0.25–0.5 mg/kg; higher doses (2 mg/kg) are anaesthetic. Side effects include salivation, increased muscle tone, and emergence delirium – all are more likely with higher doses.

Intravenous paracetamol should be considered as an opiate-sparing agent (thereby reducing the risk of missing opiate-related side effects, when multiple casualties make regular observation challenging) [6, 7].

Local anaesthetic nerve blocks will have a role at the scene to facilitate extrication, clinical intervention or packaging for transport – perhaps the most frequently used blocks in this situation will be a femoral nerve block for a fractured femur [8], or pain relief to allow a chest drain to be inserted in a conscious casualty. Blocks are more likely to be considered when evacuation is delayed and patients are held at the Casualty Clearing Station.

Inhaled analgesia has a rapid onset of action and is used substantially in pre-hospital care. Entonox (a 50:50 mixture of nitrous oxide and oxygen) has been widely used in the UK. Methoxyflurane is used extensively in Australasia for both adults and children [9], and has been formulated as a personal issue inhaler for use in combat casualty care [10].

Where cross-border or international assistance is being provided, rescuers must be aware of the relevant national laws. The use of opiates is an example where law may prohibit administration by non-doctors, or may prohibit certain brands of opiate (e.g. diamorphine).

References

1. Lynch M. Pain as the 5th vital sign. *Journal of Intravenous Nursing* 2001; **24**: 85–94.
2. Todd KH, Funk KG, Funk JP, Bonacci R. Clinical significance of reported changes in pain severity. *Annals of Emergency Medicine* 1996; **27**: 485–489.
3. Frank A, Moll J, Hort F. A comparison of three ways of measuring pain. *Rheumatology* 1982; **21**: 211–217.
4. Porter K. Ketamine in pre-hospital care. *Emergency Medicine of Journal* 2004; **21**: 351–354.
5. Svenson J, Abernathy M. Ketamine for prehospital use: new look at an old drug. *The American Journal of Emergency Medicine* 2007; **25**: 977–980.
6. Hernandez-Palazon J, Tortosa JA, Martinez-Lage JF, et al. Intravenous administration of propacetamol reduces morphine consumption after spinal fusion surgery. *Anesthesia and Analgesia* 2001; **92**: 1473–1476.
7. Peduto VA, Ballabio M, Stefanini S. Efficacy of propacetamol in the treatment of postoperative pain. Morphine-sparing effect in orthopedic surgery. *Acta Anaesthesiol Scand* 1998; **42**: 293–298.
8. McGlone R, Sadhra K, Hamer D, Pritty P. Femoral nerve block in the initial management of femoral shaft fractures. *Archives of Emergency Medicine* 1987; **4**: 163–168.

9. Chin R, Maccaskill G, Brown G, Lam L. A randomised controlled trial of inhaled methoxyflurane pain relief, in children with upper limb fracture. *Journal of Paediatrics and Child Health* 2002; **38**: A13–A14.
10. McLennan J. Is methoxyflurane a suitable battlefield analgesic? *Journal of The Royal Army Medical Corps* 2007; **153**: 111–113.

Rule 42: After the crush, remember to flush

Renal failure following crush injury has been consistently reported following earthquakes.

The principal sequelae of crush injury are rhabdomyolysis, myoglobinuria, hyperkalaemia and a metabolic acidosis. It is the myoglobinuria that results in acute renal failure (ARF).

Experience in the aftermath of an earthquake has shown that prompt, aggressive fluid resuscitation has been directly linked to the reduction of the incidence of renal failure [1]. The main aim is to ensure an effective and continuous diuresis to flush the kidneys and prevent 'clogging' of the glomerular filtration system.

Fluid resuscitation and replacement therapy that ensures a urinary output of at least 100 mL an hour is the clinical target. Volumes up to 10 litres over 24 hours have been required.

The highest published prevalence of ARF following crush injury was in the wake of the Marmara earthquake in Turkey, 1999 [2]. A total of 639 patients with ARF due to crush injury were hospitalised in 35 hospitals. Ninety-seven of the 639 patients with ARF as a result of crush injury died (15.2%). The authors concluded that patients with ARF should be rapidly transferred to undamaged peripheral general hospitals. When dialysis and intensive care are available, crush injury-related ARF patients have a lower mortality.

Following the Hanshin-Awaji earthquake (Kobe, Japan, 1995), 372 patients with crush syndrome were identified from 6107 patients admitted across 95 hospitals. ARF and mortality could be estimated from the peak serum concentration of creatine kinase, as well as the number of injured extremities [3].

Associated hyperkalaemia and lactic acidosis are treated with simple management of airway, breathing (with oxygen) and circulation with fluid replacement therapy. In addition, early use of sodium bicarbonate has a positive impact on both lactic acidosis and the treatment of myoglobinuria.

Specific intervention to treat hyperkalaemia (insulin and dextrose; nebulised ß2-agonist; sodium bicarbonate) should be used where necessary – but using calcium solutions as membrane stabilisers should be avoided as calcium ions increase the risk of muscle breakdown.

References

1. Gunal A, Celiker H, Dogukan A., et al. Early and vigorous fluid resuscitation prevents acute renal failure in the crush victims of catastrophic earthquakes. *Journal of The American Society of Nephrology* 2004; **15**: 1862–1867.
2. Erek E, Sever M, Serdengecti K., et al. An overview of morbidity and mortality in patients with acute renal failure due to crush syndrome: the Marmara earthquake experience. *Nephrology, Dialysis, Transplantation* 2002; **17**: 33–40.
3. Oda J, Tanaka H, Yoshioka T., et al. Analysis of 372 patients with crush syndrome caused by the Hanshin-Awaji earthquake. *Journal of Trauma* 1997; **42**: 470–476.

CHAPTER 8
Transport Rules

> ! Rule 43: Some T1s must go before others
>
> ! Rule 44: Beware of transferring the site of the disaster
>
> ! Rule 45: Pulse your patients to more than one receiving hospital
>
> ! Rule 46: Transfer should be a care continuum, not a care vacuum
>
> ! Rule 47: T4s leave after T1s, but before T2s
>
> ! Rule 48: Patients who are able to self-evacuate will – but they may need to be encouraged
>
> ! Rule 49: Casualties may not be evacuated in strict priority order
>
> ! Rule 50: Get patient placement right first time

Disaster Rules 1st edition. © Rob Russell, Timothy Hodgetts, Peter Mahoney and Nicholas Castle. Published 2011 by Blackwell Publishing Ltd.

Rule 43: Some T1s must go before others

When there is more than one T1 casualty for evacuation, there is a requirement for a system of sub-prioritisation.

Within the Casualty Clearing Station, patients are grouped together in priorities for treatment and packaging for transfer to definitive care. As ambulances (or helicopters) become available, the Casualty Clearing Officer and the Loading Officer will have to decide on the clinical priority for use of available resources. It is at this point where individual patient clinical needs will be used to decide on the order of transfer.

Example

Terrorist bomb. Current resource available: one paramedic ambulance. Who is to be moved first?

Patient A: Male, age 55, RR 6, P 45, SBP 170, GCS 3.

Injuries: open skull fracture with a fixed and dilated left pupil; 30% full thickness burns.

Patient B: Female, age 72, RR 24, P 110, SBP 100, GCS 15.

Injuries: bilateral below knee amputations, bleeding controlled by tourniquets.

Patient C: Female, age 29, RR 32, P130, SBP 60 (85 post fluids), GCS 14.

Injuries: penetrating abdominal injury; right-sided chest injury, suspect pneumothorax.

Patient C has a time-critical injury and requires immediate surgery; patient B also requires early surgery (and military experience is that these patients often require massive transfusion, which is defined as 10 or more units of red cells within 24 hours). Patient A has signs of a severe head injury with a Cushing response (bradycardia and hypertension) indicating raised intracranial pressure.

The order of evacuation will be a balance of the current clinical condition with an understanding of how each patient is likely to respond to treatment; this requires considerable judgement. For these three patients, when injury severity is balanced with potential survivability, the order of evacuation would be C-1st, B-2nd, A-3rd.

Rule 44: Beware of transferring the site of the disaster

The immediate aftermath of a major incident could be described as unstructured, disorganised or chaotic. The first priority for the emergency services is to overlay a structure of command and control (see Rule 1) to transform chaos into mild confusion – to achieve complete order is a tremendous and perhaps unrealistic achievement.

If casualties are effectively regulated from the scene, then the receiving hospitals have the optimal chance to cope with the surge in work load. Effective regulation means sending the right patient to the right hospital (see Rule 50) and spreading the casualty load across all the available receiving hospitals (see Rule 45).

A failure to effectively triage patients at the scene for treatment and transport, provide immediate life-saving interventions and intelligently regulate will lead to hospitals being overwhelmed – in essence, the disaster is transferred from the site to the hospital [1–6].

The Ramstein Airshow Disaster in Germany, 1988 (70 killed, about 350 seriously injured) [3, 4], is an example of poor regulation. Here, three aircraft collided mid-air and a fireball of aviation fuel engulfed the crowd. Given the wide availability of air transport assets, 120 casualties were rapidly moved to a nearby small American military hospital (about 200 beds) within the first 30 minutes. This was simply a change in the geographical location of the disaster.

The lack of pre-hospital triage and treatment compounded the incident: the nearest hospitals were filled with minor injured (T3), diverting limited resources from treating the seriously injured time-critical patients. Seriously injured patients were found at the scene unattended more than 2 hours after the incident (in addition, a bus with unattended casualties and a driver unfamiliar with the area took almost 3 hours to reach a local hospital–see Rule 35). Other compounding factors were the destruction of the on-site dedicated medical emergency helicopter, the large number of untrained volunteers, and the loss of the public address system.

At the Clapham rail crash (London, 1988), 129 patients were sent to the same hospital in less than 2 hours – despite a planned maximum number of casualties having been set at 75. This resulted in a significant over-burdening of the emergency department, particularly with regard to minor injury patients [5, 7].

There is little rationale in an urban setting of a developed health-care system to overwhelm one hospital while others wait in antic-ipation to share the load [1]. There may, of course, be occasions when only one medical facility is available, particularly in remote areas or in the military operational setting. Following an earthquake in Nepal, the British Military Hospital, Dharan, was the only intact hospital for a local population of over 100 000 people [8].

References

1. Coad N, Jones M, Byrne A, Pepperman M. The M1 air crash: the de-mands placed on anaesthetic and intensive care services of two hospitals. *Anaesthesia* 1989; **44**: 851–854.
2. Brismar B, Bergenwald L. The terrorist bomb explosion in Bologna, Italy, 1980: an analysis of the effects and injuries sustained. *Journal of Trauma* 1982; **22**: 216–220.
3. Martin T. The Ramstein airshow disaster. *Journal of the Royal Army Medical Corps* 1990; **136**: 19–26.
4. Seletz J. Flugtag-88: an army response to a MASCAL. *Military Medicine* 1990; **4**: 153–155.
5. Evans R, Perkins A. In case of emergency. *Health Service Journal* 1989; **99**: 948–950.
6. Collins S. What about us? The psychological implications of dealing with trauma following the Omagh bombing. *Emergency Nurse* 2001; **8**: 9–13.
7. Heywood-Jones I. Red alert. *Nursing Times* 1989; **85**: 16–17.
8. Guy P, Ineson N, Bailie R, Grimwood A. Operation nightingale: the role of BMH Dharan following the 1988 Nepal earthquake, some observa-tions on third world earthquake disaster relief mission. *Journal of the Royal Army Medical Corps* 1990; **136**: 7–18.

Rule 45: Pulse your patients to more than one receiving hospital

Poor regulation of casualties from the incident site to hospital can result in simply transferring the site of the emergency (see Rule 44). Where there is a choice of receiving hospitals, the seriously injured (T1 and T2 priorities) should be distributed in pulses. This provides time for emergency department assessment and initial resuscitation, before the next batch of patients arrives.

It is a false assumption that the nearest hospital will always be able to provide the quickest treatment. Busy hospitals can be by-passed in favour of others that are ready to receive casualties, but are further away – and the patients are still potentially processed faster. The judgment lies with whether the patients can tolerate the longer journey and whether appropriate clinical escorts are available.

The process of pulsing patients will be more effective if the Medical Commander and/or Loading Officer have a good local knowledge of the receiving hospitals' resuscitation capacity, and knowledge of the hospitals' specialist capabilities (so the right patient is targeted to the right hospital – see Rule 50).

An accurate bed state from each receiving hospital is essential to support decision-making and casualty regulation at the scene. The bed state must be updated regularly and ideally in real-time. A mature emergency care system will centrally coordinate information from each hospital and will provide direction for the scene health service commanders: in other words, the scene tells the coordinating headquarters the number of patients ready to be moved, their priority and any specific clinical requirements (e.g. patient is ventilated and needs medical escort; or patient is a head injury and must go direct to a neurosurgical centre). In the civilian context, this coordination will be at the Ambulance Service Headquarters; in the military context, it will be at the formation or regional command headquarters.

At some incidents, attempts to pulse patients to appropriate hospitals have been undermined by the actions of medical or ambulance staff, who failed to follow instructions [1]. Following the chain of command at major incidents, whilst not coming naturally to all healthcare professionals, is essential.

Reference

1. Malone W. Lessons to be learned from the major disaster following the civil airliner crash at Kegworth in January 1989. *Injury* 1990; **21**: 49-52.

Rule 46: Transfer should be a care continuum, not a care vacuum

The principles of evacuation are to maintain or enhance the standard of care as the patient progresses through the evacuation chain. As an example, it would be negligent (in the medical sense of the word, where there is a breach of duty of care to a patient and the patient suffers as a result) to anaesthetise, intubate and ventilate a patient in the pre-hospital setting, then hand the patient over to an ambulance crew that cannot sustain the anaesthetic in transit.

Sudden deterioration in transit will require intervention: the skills of the transport crew must match the likely risks the patient faces – for example, a patient with ischaemic chest pain should be transported by a crew who, as a minimum, can undertake basic life support and use an automated external defibrillator.

For a safe transfer with assurance that the quality of care will be sustained, tubes and lines need to be carefully secured: it may be difficult to re-site these when in transit.

- An endotracheal tube can easily be dislodged when the head and neck are moved; an end-tidal CO_2 monitor (digital reading, or colourimetric) is a valuable aid to detecting when this happens.
- Intravenous lines are easily dislodged when a patient is handled: tape them or bandage them in place – an intraosseous line offers advantage in being considerably more difficult to dislodge.
- Battery-driven monitors and ventilators must be checked to ensure they have enough life to support the mission.
- Oxygen cylinders should be checked for adequate residual content.

A simple transfer checklist can be remembered as follows:

ABC
A: Is the **A**irway secure?
B: Is **B**reathing (ventilation) adequate? Is there enough oxygen?
C: Is the **C**irculation stable? Are IV lines secured? Is there enough fluid being carried for the transfer?

NEWS
N: **N**ecessary. Has everything necessary been done?
E: **E**nough. Is there enough fluids and oxygen available?
W: **W**orking. Are all pieces of equipment working and charged?
S: **S**ecure. Are all lines and tubes secure?

Rule 47: T4s leave after T1s, but before T2s

Allocating limited resources in a major incident to a casualty who is expected to die will mean that an alternative patient who is potentially salvageable is denied treatment and may die as a result.

The T4 category is used in uncompensated major incidents when patient numbers are overwhelming, despite the deployment of extraordinary resources. T4 casualties are those whose injuries are judged to be unsalvageable: that is, the injuries are so serious that survival is unlikely even with the intervention of best medical practice [1].

T4 is not a routine triage category. Invoking the T4 category is a difficult decision that must be made by senior and experienced healthcare personnel. In the civilian context, the decision at the scene should ideally be made jointly by the senior doctor and the senior ambulance officer (the Silver Medical and Ambulance Commanders); at the hospital, the need will probably be identified by the senior emergency physician engaged with triage at the front door, but the decision should sensibly involve the senior surgeon assigning operating theatre priorities (the Surgical Triage Officer) and the doctor coordinating the hospital's major incident response (the Medical Coordinator, who may or may not be the hospital's Medical Director). In the UK military context, the category can only be authorised by the officer commanding all the pre-hospital and hospital assets in the area of operations (Commander Medical).

Understanding T4: A Case Example

A 6-year-old boy is knocked down by a car in a developed country. At the scene, he is unresponsive. There is a large, open head wound with exposed brain. The child is still breathing, rate 8/minute. There is no palpable radial or femoral pulse, but a weak and slow carotid pulse.

The actions will be:

- Call an ambulance and start resuscitation at the roadside (in some systems this may involve anaesthesia and securing a definitive airway at the roadside).
- Alert the receiving hospital and assemble the trauma team.
- Resuscitate the child on arrival at hospital and undertake a CT scan.

- Discuss the findings of the CT scan with a neurosurgeon and act accordingly.
- Potentially admit to an intensive care unit.

Somewhere in this chain the child is highly likely to die – before the ambulance arrives, during the resuscitation process, or in an intensive care unit. A developed country's trauma system would not deny this process, but when resources are limited, difficult decisions have to be made and the resources allocated intelligently.

A reluctance to instigate the T4 category is understandable. To decide not to resuscitate a patient who still has signs of life is contrary to the normal practice of the emergency services. However, failure to instigate the T4 category will lead to a greater loss of life. This is why wherever possible it should be a joint decision and the reasons fully documented: the record will offer the necessary explanation, and legal defence, during the subsequent Public Inquiry.

In a situation where there are adequate resources to offer full treatment to every casualty, there would be no T4 category – these patients would all be T1. If the T4 category has been used, but is revoked because resources become available, T4 patients who are still alive will become T1.

The triage category coupled with the availability of suitable resources dictates the order of evacuation from the scene. T1, T2 and T4 patients are likely to all require evacuation by ambulance, and this is a rate-limiting step. T1 casualties should be evacuated first – but once all T1s have been cleared from the scene, the surviving T4 casualties can be evacuated (before T2s).

Contemporary military experience has shown there is a reluctance to use 'dead' in a radio message and the dead have been labelled as 'T4'. This is unhelpful when determining the resources needed at the scene (medical transport for a casualty; or non-medical transport for a body) and when establishing the time of death within the inquiry.

Reference

1. Advanced Life Support Group. *Major Incident Medical Management and Support*. London, BMJ Publishing; 2002, 2nd edition

Rule 48: Patients who are able to self-evacuate will – but they may need to be encouraged

The natural response to a dangerous situation may be to flee, but the sudden unexpected events of a major incident may also cause people to freeze and stand still. This situation will be further aggravated if there is no obvious rally point and/or no obvious evacuation route, especially if it is dark.

A key element of patient safety and scene control is to promptly remove those casualties who can self-evacuate to a nominated point staffed by emergency personnel. This is the first element of the Triage Sieve: '*Is the casualty walking?*' (see Rule 29).

A visible rally point, such as the flashing blue lights of an emergency vehicle, will attract casualties. This can be augmented by clear instructions via a loudhailer (or public address system where available in a station, airport or stadium incident) to direct those able to walk to a safe area; triage officers, as they move forward, can also direct the walking wounded towards the Casualty Clearing Station, and the uninjured survivors can be directed separately to a safe evacuation point (over time, a Survivor Reception Centre can be established for uninjured survivors, which is managed by the Police).

Experience in urban areas is that walking wounded rapidly self-evacuate (on foot, by taxi and private transport) and present at the nearby hospitals – the first awareness of the hospital that an incident has occurred may therefore come from the public, rather than through official emergency service channels. This is the reason for retaining flexibility within the hospital's contingency plan for the hospital's major incident response to be activated by the emergency department. Ambulance Control must be informed and this can be done by the senior nurse or consultant in the emergency department: this may precede a major incident having been declared at the scene.

Rule 49: Casualties may not be evacuated in strict priority order

The order for evacuation is dictated by clinical need and the availability, capacity and suitability of transport.

Those with the highest clinical need may not be the first available for evacuation. Minor injured (T3) casualties are usually mobile and will be the first casualties to reach the Casualty Clearing Station. They invariably only require limited intervention prior to safe transfer to hospital (e.g. sling; dressing). Patients who are immobile at the point of wounding or trapped in the wreckage require to be rescued: the timeline for their evacuation includes stabilisation at point of wounding, extrication, then reassessment, treatment and packaging for transport at the Casualty Clearing Station.

T3s will often constitute the majority of casualties. The principle of transport for T3s is to bypass the nearest hospital(s): this retains capacity close to the incident for the most time-critical patients.

Following the Bradford football stadium fire, over 200 patients arrived at the local emergency department within the first hour, with the vast majority of these patients arriving via non-ambulance transfer [1]. A similar experience followed the Oklahoma City bombing where the nearest hospital was overwhelmed with casualties, many with only minor injuries [2].

Non-medical mass transport may be used for T3s (coach, bus, minibus, train). There is logic in initially observing T3s in a treatment area (presuming resources allow) as more serious injuries may unmask – the worst place for deterioration is during transport when there is no opportunity to be redirected through the evacuation system, and limited opportunity for intervention (some level of medical escort is advisable).

Factors determining when a critical patient can be moved are:
- *Capacity of the vehicle.* An emergency ambulance and an air ambulance often only have capacity for one stretcher case. There may be opportunity to take sitting patient(s) in the same vehicle as stretcher cases, in which case T2 or T3 may leapfrog a T1 who is waiting.
- *Availability of a suitable vehicle.* A helicopter may be the preferred vehicle to take a specific patient directly to a specialist unit (neurosurgery, spinal, burns). An emergency ambulance with oxygen, suction and patient monitoring will be the safe standard for some patients.

- *Availability of a suitable escort.* The standard of care initiated at the scene should be maintained or enhanced during transport to the next level of care.

While a critical patient waits for transport, others of a lower priority may be moved if suitable transport and escort are available.

The processes can be somewhat different in the military setting. A large capacity helicopter carrying a skilled medical team is the principal transport for casualty evacuation [3]. Triage and treatment will have taken place on the ground, but multiple casualties of mixed priorities will be loaded onto the helicopter. The helicopter invariably spends a very short time on the ground (2–3 minutes) to avoid becoming a target for hostile action. Triage and treatment (including advanced interventions such as rapid sequence induction of anaesthesia, surgical airway, chest drain, and administration of blood or plasma) will take place during flight, with the medical crew moving amongst the patients. This is, effectively, a Casualty Clearing Station in the air.

References

1. Sharpe D, Foo I. Management of burns in major disaster. *Injury* 1990; **21**: 41–44.
2. Emergency department impact of the Oklahoma City terrorist bomb. *Annals of Emergency Medicine* 1999; **34**: 160–167.
3. Davis P, Rickard A, Ollerton J. Determining the composition and benefit of the pre-hospital medical response team in the conflict setting. *Journal of the Royal Army Medical Corps* 2007; **153**: 269–273.

Rule 50: Get patient placement right first time

In addition to ensuring the *right order* of evacuation is followed and the *right transport* is used (see Rule 49), it is also the responsibility of the health service officers at the scene to ensure patients are sent to the *right destination* (a responsibility of the Ambulance Loading Officer, in conjunction with the Medical and Ambulance Silver Commanders).

Patients with injuries that would benefit from specialist treatment (head injuries, cardiothoracic injuries, burns, spinal injuries) are best sent direct to a hospital that has those specialist facilities. If sent to a general hospital, the patient will require secondary transport.

The exception is if the patient requires immediate life-saving intervention and the patient cannot realistically tolerate a longer journey – for example, a patient with closed head and abdominal injuries, who has signs of intra-abdominal haemorrhage that demand immediate general surgical intervention (rigid abdomen and signs of hypovolaemic shock).

Secondary transfers during a major incident are likely to pose difficulties because of the diversion of extraordinary ambulance resources to the scene.

Helicopter air ambulances have a specific utility to transfer selected casualties requiring specialist care over longer distances direct to centres of excellence, making optimum use of their enhanced reach.

CHAPTER 9
Hospital Rules

! Rule 51:   No notes, no defence

! Rule 52:   The major incident plan will not be read: use action cards

! Rule 53:   It is not all clinical: support services are a key success factor

! Rule 54:   You have longer to prepare than you think – so use the time wisely

! Rule 55:   Your first step in planning is to know your enemy

! Rule 56:   Resilience states inform capacity decisions

! Rule 57:   Nominate a dedicated major incident receiving ward

! Rule 58:   Beware of announcing a hospital stand-down as soon as the scene is clear

Disaster Rules 1st edition. © Rob Russell, Timothy Hodgetts, Peter Mahoney and Nicholas Castle. Published 2011 by Blackwell Publishing Ltd.

Rule 51: No notes, no defence

. . .or, more completely:

Good notes, good defence; poor notes, poor defence; no notes, no defence

If a drug is not prescribed, it was not given; if a decision is not recorded, it was not made; if vital signs are not charted, they were not taken.

These statements may seem obvious, but in the heat of a major incident when decisions are made quickly and personnel respond to multiple (sometimes contradicting) verbal orders, it is too easy for documentation to be incomplete. When reviewing the records retrospectively, whether to prove a good outcome or defend an adverse outcome, if it is not written down, it has to be assumed it did not happen.

All healthcare professionals are accountable for their actions. If you discussed a case with a senior colleague, write down the decision: should the patient suffer adversely it will otherwise be presumed to be your error of judgement. If you took vital signs, record them: their absence from the notes will be presumed to be your error of omission in caring for the patient. If you fail to record a resuscitation drug, you will be unable to prove the standard of care administered – or worse, you may contribute to an adverse patient outcome should a drug with cumulative side effects be inadvertently repeated (e.g. an anticoagulant).

Conversely, accurate, contemporaneous records can spare your organisation costly litigation – more importantly, good records will defend your personal reputation (remember the adage: *Reputation arrives on foot, but departs on horseback*).

This principle applies as much to the administrative decision-making process as it does to the treatment of individual patients. Logs should be maintained of all communications and decisions made. In real-time, they help the individual keep track of whether orders have been followed and actions completed. In retrospect, they serve to improve recall and provide justification during the subsequent Inquiry, but they also constitute admissible evidence. As such, they should be surrendered to the Police, after a personal copy has been made (an insurance against loss). *Do not destroy your log of a major incident.*

The generation of a clinical record on arrival at hospital takes a finite time and is usually produced after the patient has been 'booked in' with demographic details entered into a computer. This would produce a bottleneck of administration in a major incident. Instead, it is advisable to prepare documentation packs to include the emergency department record, trauma chart, imaging request form, blood product request form, haematology and biochemistry sample form, and patient wrist band. A unique series of pre-determined major incident patient numbers can be assigned. As well as making documentation easier, this also facilitates review and audit later.

Any patient attending the emergency department during the major incident should be issued with a major incident number regardless of whether they are part of the incident or not (remember, the local population will still need to be served for day-to-day emergencies such as an asthma attack, stroke, or myocardial infarction). This will prevent duplicate records and related confusion at the time of the incident. It may, however, be a challenge in retrospect to separate incident from non-incident patients – but effectiveness at the time of the incident is the paramount concern.

Rule 52: The major incident plan will not be read: use action cards

However good your planning for a major incident has been, the delivery of the plan will depend on your personnel. Despite your best efforts, some individuals will have omitted to read the plan and will have failed to take up the training – and others who have made the effort may still be unsure of their role (due to the time elapsed since their training or the stress of the situation).

Action cards are a tool to ensure that key roles are performed optimally. They are an aide memoire, listing essential tasks and important contact numbers. At a time of crisis when it is possible to be paralysed by the magnitude of the problems faced, action cards provide a structure to help order thoughts and actions.

An action card is not the major incident plan in miniature: it is a series of simple, role-specific bullet points. The target should be to limit instructions to a single side of A5 paper. On the reverse side can be key telephone numbers and, if the holder is to use a radio, a list of key call signs. The action card can be laminated and hung around the neck during an incident: if it is carried, it will be put down and misplaced.

Action cards facilitate the major incident plan to be a more manageable document to read and interpret. Instead of every employee having to read the whole document (and to identify, extract and interpret their role), there can be a short section of core principles followed by the comprehensive series of action cards. A number of appendices covering special circumstances are also valuable (incidents involving contaminated casualties; large numbers of children; burns).

An action card should be written by one of the individuals likely to fill that role (see Rule 55).

Take advantage of national and international experience from major incidents to raise awareness of the major incident plan in your own hospital. When an event is in the news and at the front of people's minds, this is a short but important opportunity to ask your staff to reflect on what they would do in the same circumstances – and to give direction on where they can find out how the hospital would respond. This campaign can be carried out by e-mail and notice-board posters for most staff, but key personnel may benefit from a telephone call or a face-to-face approach.

Rule 53: It is not all clinical: support services are a key success factor

Direct patient care will be the initial focus of the major incident response at the hospital, but the administrative and technical support services are also vital to success. Typically, plans are weighted in favour of the 'front of house' clinical staff who are geared to provide clinical care, and not the vital support staff: yet, demands on support services will be significant.

Clinical support services in initial high demand will be blood transfusion (cross match and supply of blood products), imaging (plain imaging in the resuscitation room, main X-ray department, and the operating theatre; focused abdominal sonography in trauma (FAST) ultrasound scan in the emergency department to exclude intra-abdominal free fluid; computerised tomography (CT) scan), pathology (urgent haematology and biochemistry sample processing) and sterile services (maintaining the effectiveness of the operating theatres).

Around half of the patients attending an emergency department can be expected to require radiology [1]; in one hospital following the Kegworth air crash, 409 radiological investigations were ordered and 248 units of blood were administered in the first 12 hours [2].

As the incident progresses, the roles played by hospital administrators will become more dominant in the return to normalcy.

The key administrative and clinical support elements in the hospital are:
- Hospital Control Centre
  - Overall coordination of the hospital's response
- Switchboard
  - Communication hub of the hospital
- Pathology laboratories
  - Sample processing
- Imaging
  - Plain film; ultrasound; CT; arteriography; MRI
- Sterile Services
  - Surgical instrument cleaning
- Pharmacy
  - Discharge prescriptions to facilitate casualty flow; in-patient support

- Medical stores
  - Re-supply of clinical areas with disposables
- Mortuary
  - For deaths at the hospital (deaths at the scene will be diverted to a pre-determined regional Temporary Mortuary)
- Portering
  - Move patients and urgent blood samples; to collect blood products
- Domestic/Cleaning Staff
- Medical Photography
  - Photograph wounds for clinical purposes; to photograph the dead for identification
- Catering
  - For staff, patients and visitors
- Chaplaincy and Pastoral Care
  - Welfare of patients and staff
- Hospital Executive
  - Internal support and external liaison

Administrative functions that are specific to a major incident are:

- Communication with local authorities, the Health Protection Agency, and Health Emergency Planning Advisers
- Media Liaison
  - A manager with media training should be appointed as the Media Liaison Officer
- Cancelling and reorganising planned outpatient appointments and elective surgery
- Organising return to normal hospital function and staffing
  - Return to normal function will likely take weeks (excess of patients requiring returns to the operating theatre for plastic and reconstructive procedures; impact on outpatient services to review discharges)
- Dealing with VIP visits

References

1. Hogan D, Waeckerie J, Dire D, Lillibridge S. Emergency department impact of the Oklahoma city terrorist bomb. *Annals of Emergency Medicine* 1999; **34**: 160–167.
2. Kirsh G, Learmouth D, Martindale J. The Nottingham, Leicester, Derby aircraft accident study group. *BMJ* 1989; **298**: 503–506.

Rule 54: You have longer to prepare than you think – so use the time wisely

No time spent in preparation is wasted.

Unless a major incident occurs immediately outside a hospital, or communication systems from the scene have failed, a hospital will receive warning that it is about to receive a large number of casualties. Critical patients take time to extricate and stabilise at the scene and there is often considerable time to prepare.

Notable exceptions have been when a hospital has been damaged or destroyed by an earthquake, or specifically targeted by a terrorist bomb [1]. In the military context, contemporary experience is peppered with examples of multiple casualty incidents following indirect fire onto a military base or improvised explosive devices (including suicide IEDs) close to the camp – fortunately, with all hospital staff resident adjacent to a field hospital it only takes a matter of minutes to mount a full hospital major incident response.

The actions to prepare the hospital can be structured using the CSCATTT paradigm (see Rule 1). The following are the actions for the emergency department, but a similar structure can be applied to preparation of any functional area in the hospital, whether clinical or administrative (see Rule 53).

Emergency Department (ED) Preparation

Control – a general hospital function
- Gather Hospital Control Team and establish Hospital Control Centre
- Start log of communications and actions
- Control traffic entering hospital by locking or manning doors
- Open equipment store and place external and internal signs

Command
- Start log of all communications and actions in ED
- Issue tabards (vests labelled with role) to key personnel
- Assign roles and issue Action Cards (see Rule 52)

Safety
- Establish Decontamination Facility (if required)

- Equip Mobile Emergency Response Incident Team (if needed)
- Ensure staff use basic personal protection (gloves, aprons, lead gowns)

Communication
- Doctor in charge ED to brief all ED staff
- Doctor in charge ED to brief MERIT (if needed)
- Issue radios, check call signs and batteries, carry out 'radio check' (if radios used)

Assessment
- How many casualties and what severity are anticipated?
- What non-incident patients are currently in the ED? What needs to be done for them?
- Any specialist demands? Burns/Paediatrics/Chemical/Radiation?

Triage
- Establish, equip and staff triage area
- Issue triage prompt card (if it has been prepared in planning phase)

Treatment
- Establish, equip and staff T1, T2 and T3 areas
- Set up Treatment teams
- Draw up drugs that will be needed (rapid sequence induction of anaesthesia; analgesia; antibiotics)
- Liaise with transfusion services for the requirement to prepare shock packs (O-negative red cells and AB-positive plasma for initial resuscitation of the critically hypovolaemic)
- Bring forward prepared Documentation packs (see Rule 51)
- Maintain capacity to treat concurrent non-incident sick/injured
- Be flexible in how you create additional space for casualties and personnel for Treatment teams: the casualty load may exceed your planning assumptions

Transport
- Set up Transport teams (to move patients internally)
- Transport non-incident trolley patients to wards where appropriate

- Move non-incident 'walking' patients to T3 area (if different). Inform that there will be an increased delay and encourage them to attend GP (if appropriate)

Reference

1. Hodgetts T. Lessons from the Musgrave Park Hospital bombing. *Injury* 1993; **24**: 219–221.

Rule 55: Your first step in planning is to know your enemy

If you take over the responsibility for emergency planning in your hospital or organisation, there are a number of key steps you must take:

Carry out a Risk assessment:

- What are the local threats in your area?
- What chemicals or other hazardous substances are being manufactured or transported?
- Do factories/sports arenas and other similar locations have major incident plans?
- What are the plans of other healthcare organisations in your area?

Ensure you know what your authority and line of reporting is:

- Who do you report to? This may be different to the other aspects of your job.
- What can you do/authorise/spend without more senior approval?
- **What is your budget and support?**

You will need a budget for:

- Publication of plans for each ward/department
- Signs and personnel identification tabards
- Mobile medical team equipment
- In-house education
- Communication systems

You will also require administrative support to help prepare and regularly update the plan.

Review the existing plan: Does it just need updating or do you need to start again from first principles?

Review existing national +/− regional guidance and ensure your plan meets it:

- Follow the national terminology
- Use standard major incident notification procedures
- Ensure you meet minimum requirements
- Ensure your plan is compatible with other local organisations
- Do you need to plan to provide a medical commander and/or medical team (*Medical Emergency Response Incident Team*)

Get to know your hospital: Most staff of all disciplines are familiar with only a small area of their hospital. As an emergency planner you need to widen your knowledge. Make use of others' knowledge to help you write the plan – importantly, get other personnel to write their own Action Cards (see Rule 52). Staff will know the requirements of their own roles: your job is to make sure they do it.

Set up a Major Incident Planning Committee: Ensure senior medical, nursing and managerial representation. Ensure representation from all relevant areas especially Emergency, Theatres and Anaesthetics, Critical Care and Communications.

Rule 56: Resilience States inform capacity decisions

One of the most important pieces of information to be communicated from the hospital to Silver and Gold Command is the hospital's capacity to receive casualties and deal with surge activity.

Whilst individual details (e.g. the number of ITU beds available) of the hospital's capacity may also need to be relayed, a summary picture is extremely useful as it allows the scene commanders to direct casualties to those facilities that have the most capacity and therefore are most able to deal with them. A summary picture can be communicated using the concept of *Resilience States* (RS).

As shown in Figure 9.1, as the hospital activity and casualty load rise, so does the resilience state reported by the hospital. The higher the resilience state, the less is the hospital's capacity to deal with a surge.

The critical resilience state is *RS 3* as this is the tipping point after which a further casualty load will tip a hospital into *RS 4*, or *Major Incident Declared*.

The resilience state concept was developed for use in military hospitals on operations as a way of conveying to senior commanders the level of activity in a field hospital, thereby allowing military operations to be planned against capacity. In the UK, most, if not all, NHS Hospitals are permanently operating at *RS 3* by the definitions given.

Experience in the military setting does cloud the use of such a concept. If a major incident is declared at the hospital, it is a clear message to commanders that other activity generating further casualties will exceed the available medical capacity. The implication of declaring a major incident at a field hospital must, therefore, be very carefully considered if the operational imperative is to be maintained.

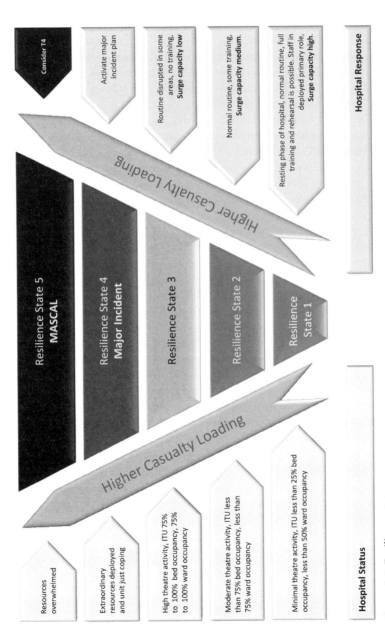

Hospital Response

Consider T4

Activate major incident plan

Routine disrupted in some areas, no training. **Surge capacity low**

Normal routine, some training. **Surge capacity medium.**

Resting phase of hospital, normal routine, full training and rehearsal is possible. Staff in deployed primary role. **Surge capacity high.**

Higher Casualty Loading

Resilience State 5
MASCAL

Resilience State 4
Major Incident

Resilience State 3

Resilience State 2

Resilience
State 1

Higher Casualty Loading

Hospital Status

Resources overwhelmed

Extraordinary resources deployed and unit just coping

High theatre activity, ITU 75% to 100% bed occupancy, 75% to 100% ward occupancy

Moderate theatre activity, ITU less than 75% bed occupancy, less than 75% ward occupancy

Minimal theatre activity, ITU less than 25% bed occupancy, less than 50% ward occupancy

Figure 9.1 Resilience states.

121

Rule 57: Nominate a dedicated major incident receiving ward

Using a single ward to receive casualties from a major incident provides a number of advantages:
- Concentration of medical, nursing and supporting (porters, pharmacist, physiotherapist) resources
- Facilitates intra-incident and post-incident ward rounds
- Simplifies documentation
- Facilitates casualty identification and reunion with relatives
- Aids continuing assessment of the clinical situation
- Simplifies VIP and media management post-incident

The major incident receiving ward should be identified within the planning process. A secondary receiving ward should also be identified in case of overflow. Depending on the threat assessment, further wards may be identified and supplementary plans made for 'surge management'. These plans may include using mothballed wards; using Day Surgery Unit(s); creating capacity in the hospital gym (and other available non-clinical areas); or erecting temporary shelters. The Day Surgery Unit has a particular value – it will be empty overnight and at weekends, and even if occupied during the day, the pre-operative and post-operative patients can easily be discharged, while peri-operative patients will quickly recover.

The staff on the major incident receiving ward must be aware of the ward's change in role during a multiple casualty incident and be involved in writing their action plan. One of the most crucial components is the process for clearing the ward to receive casualties from the incident. Most hospitals operate at high bed occupancy rates and this will be a challenge.

One way of achieving this is to require other wards to identify two beds to take patients from the major incident receiving ward. Most wards will be able to do this. The receiving ward can then pulse patients to the other wards in a pre-determined order. This process can be practised easily without moving any patients as part of major incident exercising.

Rule 58: Beware of announcing a hospital stand-down as soon as the scene is clear

The stand-down from a major incident will be phased. When the scene is reported clear of casualties, do not relax at the hospital. The activity to process existing patients may be intense, and there may be further patients in transit to the receiving hospitals.

The recovery phase at the hospital will begin in the ED. There is an imperative for the ED to return to normal activity rapidly, as the local population needs to be served for the daily routine of medical emergencies (angina, asthma, convulsions, stroke etc.), which will not have ceased simply because there is a major incident.

A period to clean and restock the ED is required. Immediately after this the process of debriefing and defusing can start with a quick operational debrief: gather all the department staff together, tell them they have done well, seek immediate feedback on important sticking points, and ask for a written brief from team leaders within 48 hours. It is important to concentrate on the positives: this is a time when team cohesion is strongly built.

The recovery phase will stage through the rest of the hospital depending on the nature of the incident and the type of casualties. Incidents involving medical or chemical casualties, for example, would not place a demand on the operating theatre capacity, but would strain ITU and ward beds.

The planning of the recovery phase by hospital administrators is vital and must start whilst the major incident is in progress. All areas of the hospital will need to return to normal working patterns. New outpatient appointments and revised operating lists will need to be organised for those missed as a result of the major incident: patients from the major incident do not take absolute priority and the clinical needs of the entire patient population need to be prioritised. All patients discharged home from the ED during the incident should also have a planned review to ensure that no injuries have been missed.

Contemporary experience from field hospitals is the major incident cycle (*plan–prepare–respond–recover*) is repeated regularly. People need to know they have done the right thing, or processes need to be adapted quickly, as the next incident that demands a pan-hospital response may only be a few days away (dealing with a series of troops in contact incidents, roadside bombs, and suicide IEDs means a field hospital is used to gearing up into its major incident response). The capacity of a field hospital to respond to a close series of major incidents is maintained because of the ability to rapidly clear in-patients to receiving hospitals in the home nation, after the initial life-saving interventions have been undertaken.

CHAPTER 10
Mass Gathering Rules

! Rule 59: Casualty numbers at a mass gathering are entirely predictable

! Rule 60: Panic is contagious – beware the stampede

! Rule 61: Crowds produce friction: pre-position your assets

! Rule 62: Following a crowd disturbance, separate your casualties

Disaster Rules 1st edition. © Rob Russell, Timothy Hodgetts, Peter Mahoney and Nicholas Castle. Published 2011 by Blackwell Publishing Ltd.

Rule 59: Casualty numbers at a mass gathering are entirely predictable

The majority of major incidents are not predicted – otherwise, preventative measures or steps to ameliorate the number of casualties could have been taken. By extrapolation, in most situations, resources will not be in place at 'ground zero' when the incident occurs. Most major incidents therefore start uncompensated until extraordinary resources can be mobilised.

The exception is a mass gathering, where casualty numbers can be predicted by the nature and type of event; whether the crowd is sitting or standing, static or mobile; the duration of the event; and the presence or absence of alcohol [1]. Local knowledge, previous experience and liaison with the other emergency services, especially the Police, will allow for a reasonable forecast of potential casualty numbers.

This knowledge is key in the planning of medical, security and stewarding assets at a mass gathering with the aim to comfortably treat the projected number of expected casualties. This gives the ability to deal with a minor or moderate unexpected increase without requiring an 'extraordinary response'. Following the Hillsborough disaster, Lord Justice Taylor identified minimum medical and stewarding levels required for mass gathering events and it is within this framework that an event should be staffed in the UK [2].

The unexpected should always be anticipated and certain eventualities can be planned for, such as an exceptionally hot day. However, the truly unpredictable event that generates mass casualties (a fire, structural collapse, crowd stampede to escape the rain, or terrorist incident) will require an extraordinary local response and potential declaration of a major incident.

The availability of on-site medical facilities should enable an immediate response to a major incident at a mass gathering. A contingency plan to pre-assign roles and pre-position both staff and equipment will be instrumental in gaining early Command and Control as well as instigating prompt Triage, Treatment and Transport (see Rule 1).

References

1. Cooke M, Hodgetts T. The largest mass gathering. *BMJ* 1999; **318**: 957–958.
2. Lord Justice Taylor. *Final Report into the Hillsborough Stadium Disaster*. London, HMSO; 1990.

Rule 60: Panic is contagious – beware the stampede

The behaviour of a large crowd and the individuals within it is often unpredictable and may be potentially uncontrollable should panic set in. The normal instinct is to stay with familiar routes and this typically results in the public trying to evacuate via the same route they entered unless they are clearly directed to evacuate via a different route.

There is a potential conflict of interest between the need to control movement, especially entrance to mass gatherings, and the ability to allow large numbers to leave at speed. The former is important both on safety grounds and to prevent unauthorised or unpaid entry, but may adversely affect emergency evacuation unless an agreed and practised evacuation plan is in place.

A key design element regarding the flow of the public at a mass gathering is to allow rapid dispersal at the end of the event and prompt evacuation. This is particularly important at older venues where such considerations may not have been part of the original design.

The identification of 'pinch-points' or other areas where congestion can readily occur will focus attention on how stewards must control these areas optimally. Mobile medical assets should be positioned to cover exit points and to follow the crowds as they disperse (see Rule 61). This should take place even when the event has gone off without a hitch. This will provide prompt on-site medical cover should it be required, as well as providing commentary/information should incidents arise.

Rule 61: Crowds produce friction: pre-position your assets

Planning the medical response and where assets will be located takes thought and experience to avoid pitfalls. Any movement through a large crowd, either with or against the flow of crowd movement will be significantly slower than travelling the same distance when the crowd is not present. This must be considered when carrying out appreciations prior to the event.

Medical planners also need to envisage the potential crowd flows at different times during the event. Liaison with the event management team will gain valuable insights into how the event will be run. In particular, identifying peak times of crowd movement (e.g. to bars, food outlets and toilets during half-time at a football match) will be important as the response to medical emergencies will be slower during these periods.

Pre-positioning and deployment of mobile assets that move with the crowd will increase the speed of response as will careful consideration of the position of first-aid posts. Prompt responses to medical emergencies as well as medical assistance during localised evacuations can minimise the risk of loss of local containment and the associated risk of degeneration into a full-blown major incident.

The concept of *friction* is further extended in the military context. The famous nineteenth century military strategist, Carl von Clausewitz, described friction as the sum of all the minor factors that together lowered performance and undermined achieving the objective [1]. Encapsulating this concept, he identified, 'Everything in war is very simple, but the simplest thing is very difficult.'

In the context of a major incident, *friction* in this extended sense may be anticipated from the following:
- Any difficulty in identifying who is in command and/or the location of a service's command post (see Rule 13).
- Inadequate communication between those experiencing difficulties (at the point of care delivery) and the tactical decision makers (see Rule 19) – this is the *power to truth* distance. This may be a lack of initiative to pass the relevant information, or a lack of available process (inadequate communication tools).
- Inadequate physical resources (number and/or skill mix of staff; clinical equipment, drugs and re-supply of disposables; shelter; transport for patients).

- Inadequate security, necessary to control non-essential personnel (public, media, volunteers).

Reference

1. Howard M. *Clausewitz: A Very Short Introduction.* Oxford, Oxford University Press; 2002.

Rule 62: Following a crowd disturbance, separate your casualties

There are some planned mass gatherings where the potential for crowd disturbance requires specific consideration, not just at the scene but also at the receiving hospitals. Examples of these are sporting occasions with opposing teams that have a history of violence between supporters; or some political rallies; and marches (e.g. the marching season of the Orange Order in Northern Ireland, with a particular flashpoint for confrontation in Drumcree).

In such circumstances, the choice of receiving hospitals may be predetermined, with opposition elements segregated – presuming that the clinical needs of patients (in particular, any specialist needs that may be regionally proved) can still be met. This is an opportunity to avoid the risk of continuing violence as patients, with their friends and relatives, relocate to the hospitals.

A further burden to the Police will be the allocation of additional officers to hospitals to defuse confrontation. Occasionally, the need to allocate a separate hospital to receive injured police officers and other security and rescue personnel will also need to be given consideration.

The limited capacity of a field hospital often means that there is no opportunity to separate enemy forces from coalition soldiers on separate wards. From a medical perspective, all patients are treated in a humanitarian way according to clinical need – but the sensitivity of juxtaposed patients from opposing forces cannot be ignored. Enemy forces will be guarded, and curtains or screens can be used to at least create a visible barrier.

CHAPTER 11
Special Incident Rules

! Rule 63:	Casualty decontamination is a healthcare priority	
! Rule 64:	Consider your local utilities when planning for mass unconventional casualties	
! Rule 65:	Unconventional incidents require unconventional assistance	
! Rule 66:	With hazardous materials, presume the worst and respond accordingly	
! Rule 67:	Think once, think twice, think HAZMAT	
! Rule 68:	The 4 I's of CBRN exposure	
! Rule 69:	Triage is expanded for CBRN casualties	
! Rule 70:	A simple change in position can save lives	
! Rule 71:	The solution to pollution is dilution	
! Rule 72:	When decontaminating, prevent recontamination	
! Rule 73:	A requirement for dexterity is a recipe for difficulty	
! Rule 74:	When in doubt, wash it out – still in doubt, chop it out	
! Rule 75:	Toxidrome recognition is all in the eyes	

Disaster Rules 1st edition. © Rob Russell, Timothy Hodgetts, Peter Mahoney and Nicholas Castle. Published 2011 by Blackwell Publishing Ltd.

! Rule 76:   Patients present with biological syndromes, not laboratory diagnoses

! Rule 77:   Sepsis is the final fatal biological syndrome

! Rule 78:   Time–distance–shielding: the three principles of radiation protection

! Rule 79:   The radiation may kill in years, but the tension kills in minutes

Rule 63: Casualty decontamination is a healthcare priority

It has been an enduring historical misconception that the fire service is adequately equipped and prepared to provide on-site decontamination facilities at a chemical, biological, radiation or nuclear (CBRN) incident for casualties, uninjured survivors, rescue workers, and their vehicles and equipment. As a result, until recently, very few ambulance services or hospitals had the equipment and training for casualty decontamination [1].

With the exception of specialist fire appliances, individual fire engines are equipped to decontaminate crew members that have been exposed to chemicals. This is achieved via high-volume, high-pressure water delivered as a spray. This approach is designed to decontaminate fire service personnel wearing protective clothing and is probably inappropriate for dealing with the uninjured, let alone the symptomatic requiring treatment.

Fire personnel can improvise a low-pressure, high-volume system for mass decontamination, but this will be less effective than the 'wash, rinse, wash' technique and if clothing is not removed and bagged, there is a risk of recontamination (see Rules 71 and 72).

A large-scale CBRN incident will require effective mass decontamination following initial triage. This will demand the early involvement of healthcare professionals trained in triage, decontamination and emergency care procedures, who must be confident to undertake these interventions while wearing specialist protective clothing. Substantial progress has been made in recent years in providing the equipment and training required within the health services, although the preparedness across the UK is not consistent.

Reference

1. Saunders P, Ward G. Decontamination of chemically contaminated casualties: implications for the health service and a regional strategy. *Pre-Hospital Immediate Care* 2000; **4**: 122–125.

Rule 64: Consider your local utilities when planning for mass unconventional casualties

The terrorist attacks in Tokyo, New York and London have demonstrated the potential for a large number of casualties that may be a result of CBRN agents. This is a situation that, in the absence of anticipation and careful preparation, could rapidly overwhelm even the most established healthcare system.

A major concern of planners is the management of a large cohort of exposed and contaminated walking survivors, who are either uninjured or who have minor injuries. At a non-CBRN incident, the minor injured (T3s) will often self-evacuate from the immediate area of hazard, can be gathered together and moved by mass transport (bus, coach, train). If decontamination is needed prior to evacuation, there may be significant on-site delays prior to transport. Because this group is by definition mobile, containing them at the scene maybe difficult and may generate public disorder.

The process of decontamination is simple and is based on the 'wash, rinse, wash' process designed to remove chemical soiling, and specifically particles. For this to be effective, access to warm water and a weak detergent solution is required (see Rule 71). In a mass casualty situation, the fire service are capable of providing high-volume, low-pressure water spray systems (cold, dirty water), but this is less than ideal. A planning consideration is how else can high-volume, low-pressure *warm* water decontamination be improvised?

One option is the transport of uninjured survivors and casualties with very minor injuries to municipal showers, such as at local swimming pools. Under supervision of healthcare providers, self-decontamination can be undertaken with warm water and detergent, as well as with an element of privacy.

The disadvantages of this approach are that it will be possible with only a limited number of chemical agents; the vehicle(s) providing transport will need decontamination, as will the premises used; and there must be safe removal of any contaminated water – even significantly diluted pollutants may be inappropriate for disposal into the normal sewage system, and environmental damage from leaks into the river and groundwater systems must be avoided.

Rule 65: Unconventional incidents require unconventional assistance

Although traditional emergency personnel will still be at the forefront of any response to a major incident involving potential chemical or biological agents, the specialised nature of such incidents is such that other organisations will also need to be mobilised. This is not only to deal with existing and potential casualties, but also to prevent escalation of the incident, control environmental damage and help restore normality.

Agencies and individuals required to provide advice and support to commanders as well as incident monitoring are:

Directors of Public Health
Toxicologists
Microbiologists
Environmental health officials
Local Council officials
Water and sewage officials
Civil engineers
Military personnel

In large-scale incidents, local general practitioners, pharmacies and community nurses may be needed to help treat those affected but not requiring hospital treatment.

Systems to identify key personnel as well as processes to allow pharmacists and nurses to provide specific treatments should be considered and put in place within the planning phase. Such systems should be flexible and support the response to any chemical/biological incident, not just those associated with acts of terrorism. This has been demonstrated by the national and international response to the SARS and H1N1 (swine influenza) viruses.

Rule 66: With hazardous materials, presume the worst and respond accordingly

And **Better to scale down from a position of strength, than scale up from a position of weakness**

Major chemical incidents are rare (Bhopal, 1985). However, in the presence of an expansive chemical industry and the credible risk of plant incidents (fire, explosion, leakage) and incidents during transport, it is important that emergency personnel responding to a chemical incident presume the worst and then step down as required [1, 2].

Emergency personnel responding to incidents may or may not be initially aware of what agent has been released. With this lack of information, it is difficult to gauge how the agent may interact with the exposed population and the number and severity of casualties. Therefore, an 'all-hazards approach' is undertaken (see Rule 1). For personal safety, Chemical Personal Protective Equipment (CPPE) is worn until more information is available or a dynamic risk assessment (DRA) has been made [3].

The principal aim at a major incident involving chemicals is to contain casualties and uninjured survivors at the incident site and decontaminate them prior to transfer to hospital.

Hospital staff must be able to provide effective decontamination at the hospital 'front door' as casualties may also self-present to a local emergency department (ED) (although not necessarily the closest) or their primary care physician. One of the most important tasks of the pre-hospital response is the notification of *all* local hospitals that an incident has happened. When this does not happen, the first indication a hospital has of a significant hazardous material (HazMat) incident is the presentation of casualties at ED. Table 11.1 highlights this, showing the methods of transport used by casualties during the Tokyo Sarin attack (1995) to one of the receiving hospitals [4].

Major radiation incidents are also rare (Chernobyl, 1986). Minor radiation incidents do, however, occur and often in relation to the transport and spillage of radioisotopes used in medicine – typically, there would be no radiation casualties, or very limited casualties. Any spillage of radiation that produces even limited casualties is likely to produce a considerable media response.

Table 11.1 Patient transport to St Luke's International
Hospital in Tokyo, Japan, after sarin gas release [4]

Mode of arrival	Number of cases	(%)
On foot	174	(34.9)
Taxi	120	(24.1)
Car (passing Good Samaritans)	67	(13.5)
Car (Tokyo Metro Fire Department)	64	(12.9)
Ambulance	35	(7.0)
Police patrol car	7	(1.4)
Others	31	
Total	498	

References

1. Cone D, Davidson S. Hazardous materials preparedness in the emergency department. *Pre-Hospital Emergency Care* 1997; **1**: 85–90.
2. Totenhofer R, Kierce M. It's a disaster: emergency departments' preparation for a chemical incident. *Accident and Emergency Nursing* 1999; **7**: 141–147.
3. Saunders P, Ward G. Decontamination of chemically contaminated casualties: implications for the health service and a regional strategy. *Pre-Hospital Immediate Care* 2000; **4**: 122–125.
4. Okumura T, Suzuki K, Fukuda A, Kohama A, Takasu N, Ishimatsu S, Hinohara S. The Tokyo subway Sarin attack disaster management, Part 1: community emergency response. *Academic Emergency Medicine* 1998; **5**: 613–617.

Rule 67: Think once, think twice, think HAZMAT

A CBRN (chemical, biological, radiation and nuclear) incident is defined as an incident involving hazardous materials (HazMat) that have been deliberately released [1].

The number and mode of presentation of the casualties exposed to HazMat, whether due to accidental or deliberate (CBRN) release, may be the only initial clue that there are specific safety implications for those responding to the incident (Table 11.2).

To prevent escalation of the incident (i.e. further avoidable casualties including those from the emergency services), it is imperative that first responders are alert to the possibility of HazMat material release, even if the initial assessment does not identify an obvious source.

In all incidents where there are multiple casualties and the cause is not known, HazMat must be considered and the necessary safety precautions taken.

Additional clues to the nature of the HazMat agent will be apparent from the symptom cluster and pattern of physical signs (see Rules 68, 75 and 76).

Table 11.2 Steps 1-2-3

Step 1	ONE casualty	Respond as NORMAL Always consider any unusual presentation
Step 2	TWO casualties	Respond, but approach with CAUTION Report on arrival and update Control
		Consider all options
		DO NOT APPROACH Withdraw
Step 3	THREE or more casualties	Contain Report Isolate yourself and send for specialist help

If any incident results in emergency responders becoming unwell: *manage as step 3*

Reference

1. Health Protection Agency. CBRN incidents: Clinical management and health protection. London, 2005. Accessible at: HPA website: www.hpa.org.uk.

Rule 68: The 4 I's of CBRN exposure

The effects of CBRN agents can be summarised using the 4 I's.

When assessing a casualty with potential hazardous material exposure, consider clinical symptom and sign patterns and clusters to indicate the likely cause. This should be cross-referenced with supporting scientific data from the scene using intelligence, as well as Detection, Identification and Monitoring (DIM) equipment.

The 4 I's are:

Intoxication (chemical; biological, toxins).
Infection (biological, live agents).
Irradiation (radiological/nuclear).
Injuries (associated trauma).

The signs are summarised in Table 11.3.

The onset of symptoms depends upon the latency of the agent involved (see Figure 11.1).

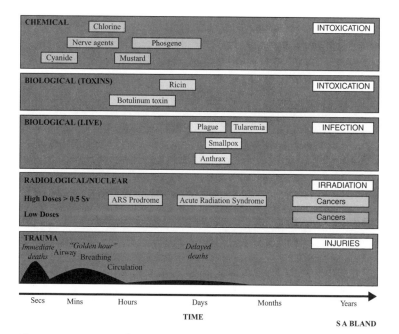

Figure 11.1 CBRN and trauma effects with time.

Table 11.3 Summary of the 4 Is

	Chemical (Intoxication)	Biological (late) (Infection)	Radiological (Irradiation)	Trauma (Injuries)
Clinical	Change in pupils	Pyrexia	Nausea	Signs of penetrating trauma
	Respiratory distress	Purpuric rash	Vomiting	Bruising
	Excessive secretions	Descending paralysis	Diarrhoea	Gross deformity
	Cyanosis in absence of trauma	Biological syndrome	Erythema	Pain
	Fitting in absence of trauma Non-thermal burns	presentation	(high doses only)	Signs of complications incl. tension pneumothorax and hypovolemia
Scientific	Chemical agent monitors – beware false positives	Environmental polymerase chain reaction (PCR) if obvious biological sample	Contamination monitor	Nil
	Mass spectroscopy	Biological sampling from patient (late)	Radiation dosimeter	

Trauma and the lethal chemical agents are likely to present earlier than the live biological agents and low-dose radiation. For this reason, the early stages of CBRN incident management should focus on the management of life-threatening injuries and the neutralisation and treatment of lethal chemical agents, with decontamination as a concurrent process (see Rule 73).

Rule 69: Triage is expanded for CBRN casualties

Triage is part of the generic CSCATTT 'all-hazards approach' to a major incident (see Rule 1).

The principles and key decisions pertinent to CBRN casualty management need to be related to this framework, in particular:

- Prioritisation of casualties for decontamination and/or treatment
- Recognition of the risk of secondary contamination
- Recognition of the risk of secondary infection
- Specific assessment and treatment of chemical, biological and radiological casualties
- Assessment and treatment of associated conventional traumatic injuries

The CSCATTT framework can be expanded to take account of these additional requirements. This can be summarised in Figure 11.2 using **TCI** instead of a single **T** for Triage:

- Command
- Safety
- Communication
- Assessment
- Triage
  - **T**riage category for treatment and decontamination?
  - **C**ontaminated or **C**ontagious?
  - **I**ntoxicated/**I**nfected/**I**rradiated/**I**njured?
- Treatment
- Transport

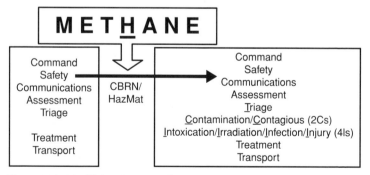

Figure 11.2 Modifying CSCATTT for CBRN.

Rule 70: A simple change in position can save lives

A number of industrial chemicals and chemical warfare agents cause loss of consciousness with resultant potential airway compromise. While this may be reversible (over time, or with the administration of an antidote), there may be limited on-scene medical or rescue personnel to provide airway skills. An example is the use of an incapacitating agent (presumed opiate gas) at the Moscow theatre siege (2002; >300 killed, >700 injured), resulting in hundreds of cases requiring ventilatory support.

As part of the modification to the Triage Sieve in a chemical environment, patients with their airway at risk should be immediately rolled into the '$3/4$-prone' position to minimise aspiration of stomach contents, and to maintain the airway. The rescuer should complete the labelling of the patient before moving on to the next casualty.

Use of the $3/4$-prone position may optimise the number of potential survivors, whilst freeing up clinicians or non-medical rescuers to provide the most for the most – note, the $3/4$-prone position places the casualty on their side, but is more stable than the 'recovery position' from which a casualty can roll more easily onto their back.

Unconscious patients should not be laid on their back following chemical exposure. There was a criticism of the rescue method following the Moscow theatre siege where the incapacitating agent resulted in hypoxic brain injuries due to unprotected airways.

Rule 71: The solution to pollution is dilution

Decontamination may be a life-saving intervention, especially in cases of gross chemical contamination. However, in some cases of chemical exposure, decontamination may not be needed – this includes incidents involving gases and non-persistent vapour, although removal of clothing may still be required (see Rule 73). Examples of non-persistent gases are hydrogen cyanide and carbon monoxide.

The process for decontamination should include the following [1]:

• Remove from contaminated (hazardous) area
• Administer life-saving interventions
• Remove clothing
• Rinse any areas of obvious, gross, liquid contamination
• Rinse– wipe–rinse
• Confirm adequate decontamination

The use of wet decontamination with warm water and detergent is based upon the risk assessment of the supervising Incident Officer.

Warm water is suggested to minimise hypothermia while preventing increased percutaneous absorption due to hot water increasing skin blood flow.

Detergent may help break up some viscous substances: however, it also provides a useful visual reference for the adequacy of the rinse process.

Wet decontamination works in two ways. Firstly, the water physically removes the contaminant and dilutes it; secondly, for chemical hazards, water may also deactivate the hazard by hydrolysis. In some cases, hydrolysis may be more effective at higher pH values, and for this reason weak bleach solution (hypochlorite, 0.5%) is sometimes recommended for the traditional chemical warfare agents, such as mustard and the nerve agents, if detected.

Decontamination of casualties is usually the responsibility of health services and should be started as soon as possible on scene. Additional resources may be required at the emergency department to deal with 'self-presenters'. The UK Fire and Rescue Services are equipped to provide mass decontamination of the uninjured survivors. The greatest challenge is the time required to set up mobile decontamination showers with the associated risk of casualty dispersal leading to the loss of control.

It is important that any delay in establishing decontamination does not delay other life-saving interventions, including basic airway and trauma management as well as early antidote administration.

Reference

1. Home Office. *Decontamination of People Exposed to Chemical, Biological, Radiological or Nuclear (CBRN) Substances or Material.* London; 2004, 2nd edition. Accessible at: http://security.homeoffice.gov.uk/news-publications/publication-search/cbrn-guidance/decon-people?view=Standard&pubID=402260.

Rule 72: When decontaminating, prevent recontamination

Following exposure to nuclear, biological or chemical agents, exposed clothing absorbs and holds contaminants. The clothing may then 'off-gas' and cause further exposure to the casualty or emergency responder. The removal of external clothing removes upwards of 80% of external contamination [1].

To minimise the risk of recontamination, off-gassing and continuing exposure of the casualty, the clothing should be carefully removed and placed into clear plastic bags. Contaminated clothing, as well as the plastic bags, should only be handled by staff wearing appropriate protection. All contaminated clothing should be 'double-bagged'. Essential personal property (such as house keys and glasses) should be separated, decontaminated and returned to the casualty.

Clothes removal process (conscious, mobile casualty):
• Instruct individual to stand with arms and legs apart
• Cut clothing along seams
• Remove clothing without pulling 'inside-out' or by pulling over the patient's head

Careful removal of clothing is of paramount importance, regardless of the degree of exposure or symptoms of casualties. It is of equal importance for the safe decontamination of uninjured survivors, especially in the presence of gross liquid contamination.

When mass decontamination is required, prompt removal of clothing is important – but ethnic and sex considerations should be factored into the mass decontamination plan. In addition, the provision of temporary clothing once decontamination has taken place is important: single-use paper suits may be an acceptable option.

Reference

1. Health Protection Agency. *CBRN Incidents: Clinical Management and Health Protection*. London, 2005. Accessible at: HPA website: www.hpa.org.uk.

Rule 73: A requirement for dexterity is a recipe for difficulty

Severely affected casualties following a CBRN incident may not survive without life-saving interventions performed concurrently with on-scene decontamination.

These life-saving interventions include:
* Control of catastrophic haemorrhage
* Basic airway management
* Early antidote administration
* Decompression of tension pneumothorax
* Fluid replacement

Traditional airway and vascular access skills involve fine motor movement, which is significantly degraded by personal protective equipment required in a chemical environment. In addition to loss of fine motor skills, vision is impaired by the use of respiratory protection.

The adaptation to use less dexterous interventions results in a higher success rate and faster skill completion. Endotracheal intubation can in the initial phase be replaced by a laryngeal mask airway which is faster to insert although not a definitive airway [1]. Intraosseous intravascular access is a viable option to peripheral venous cannulation for both fluid and antidote treatment while wearing PPE [2, 3].

Practical skills should be practised in simulated emergencies to allow staff to learn how to adapt their practice within this semi-permissive environment. A learning effect can be demonstrated with emergency skills when repeated within a 'training environment'.

References

1. Goldik Z, Burstein Y, Eden A, Ben-Abraham R. Airway management by physicians wearing anti-chemical warfare gear: comparison between laryngeal mask airway and endotracheal intubation. *European Journal of Anaesthesiology* 2002; **19**: 166–169.
2. Ben-Abraham R, Gur I, Vater Y, Weinbroum AA. Intraosseous emergency access by physicians wearing full protective gear. *Academic Emergency Medicine* 2003; **10**: 1407–1410.
3. Vardi A, Berkenstadt H, Levin I, Bentencur A, Ziv A. Intraosseous vascular access in the treatment of chemical warfare casualties assessed by advanced simulation: proposed alteration of treatment protocol. *Anesthesia and Analgesia* 2004; **98**: 1753–1758.

Rule 74: When in doubt, wash it out – still in doubt, chop it out

There are naturally concerns for responders dealing with contaminated wounds during a chemical, biological or radiation incident. The most important intervention is the removal of external chemical contamination in parallel with life-saving interventions.

Any chemical agents that are potent enough to be a secondary hazard to medical responders treating a contaminated wound are likely to have already have been fatal to the patient. Any contaminated foreign bodies that are removed should be immediately sealed in a container for disposal or forensic analysis.

Initial management of wound contamination is irrigation with copious amounts of water (wound washout). Other neutralising agents have also been suggested, but most are unlikely to provide any additional benefit and may lead to delayed healing.

Biological toxins such as ricin or botulinum may be incorporated into improvised explosive devices: consider particularly if there is contaminated shrapnel present. In this situation, surgical debridement is the principal component of wound decontamination [1].

With either chemical or biological toxin poisoning, some systemic absorption may already have taken place through the wound and any subsequent effect may need to be treated.

The same principles apply to radiological contamination and shrapnel. Care should be taken once the fragments have been removed to ensure that any further radiation exposure is limited by the principles of time, distance and shielding.

Reference

1. Cooper GJ, Ryan JM, Galbraith KA. The surgical management in war of penetrating wounds contaminated with chemical warfare agents. *Journal of the Royal Army Medical Corps* 1994; **140**: 113–118.

Rule 75: Toxidrome recognition is all in the eyes

During a chemical incident, there are number of ways to identify the type of agent involved. Even though in many cases the mainstay of treatment is supportive management, early diagnosis is important for the few chemical agents that have antidotes available. Fortunately, a number of these agents have specific toxidromes that aid diagnosis, and these agents include the following:

• Nerve agents (organophosphate)
• Cyanide
• Fentanyl derivative (opiates)
• Methaemaglobin formers

A toxidrome is a collection of physical signs due to a toxic, usually chemical, agent. Emergency responders should be able to diagnose some of these syndromes (Table 11.4) by assessing the following:

• Eyes
• Respiratory pattern
• Skin colour and perspiration
• Secretions
• Other associated features

   Eye signs can be particularly helpful as the presence of pinpoint pupils can focus the diagnosis on a very limited group of agents (nerve agent, opiate), both with antidotes available (Figure 11.3).

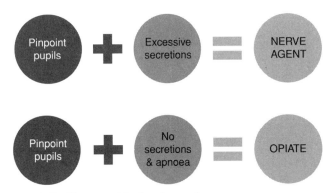

Figure 11.3 Toxidromes with pinpoint pupils.

Table 11.4 Toxidrome recognition summary

	CBRN quick look							
	Nerve agent	Cyanide	Methaemoglobin	Pulmonary agents	Mustard/lewisite	Botulism	Atropine	Opiate
EYES	Pinpoint	N/dilated	N	N	N/red	Dilated	Dilated	Pinpoint
Respiration	↑↑	↑↑/↓	↑	↑↑	↑	↓	N/↑	↓
Skin	Sweaty	Pink or cyanosed	Cyanosed	Normal or cyanosed	Erythema	Dry	Dry	N
Secretions	↑↑	N	N	↑	N/↑	↓	↓	N
Other	Fasciculation Fitting	Sudden onset	Chocolate blood		Mustard (delayed)	↓ paralysis, no CNS effects	CNS effects	CNS effects

Rule 76: Patients present with biological syndromes, not laboratory diagnoses

The Centre for Disease Prevention and Control (CDC) produces a list of significant biological threats based upon lethality, transmissibility and infectivity. These are graded into three classes (Table 11.5). The early identification of an organism is important so that definitive management may be started.

However, a patient will not likely present with a diagnosis of inhalation anthrax, plague or influenza (except in established outbreaks, when the informed patient has a high index of suspicion). Patients will present instead with a syndrome that may suggest a causative agent. Definitive diagnosis of the specific biological agent will depend on the history, clinical examination and initial investigation. This will lead to a provisional diagnosis until it has a laboratory confirmation.

Patients are likely to have an initial prodromal syndrome of flu-like symptoms including fever, arthralgia and lethargy. There are then six associated syndromes that may suggest the causative agent. These six syndromes are shown in Figure 11.4 with their typical causative agents.

It should be noted that some organisms, such as *Bacillus anthracis* (anthrax) present in a number of ways.

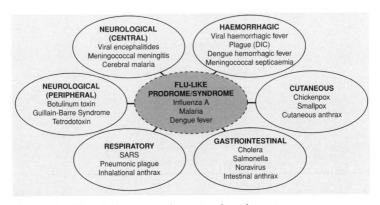

Figure 11.4 Biological agents and associated syndromes.

Table 11.5 Classification of biological agents

Class A	Class B	Class C
Properties include: High lethality High infectivity Person-to-person spread	Properties include: Moderate lethality Moderate infectivity Public health interest Possible person-to-person spread	Properties include: Emerging threat Potential for deliberate release
Anthrax (*Bacillus anthracis*) Botulism (*Clostridium botulinum* toxin) Plague (*Yersinia pestis*) Smallpox (*Variola major*) Tularemia (*Francisella tularensis*) Viral hemorrhagic fevers (filoviruses [e.g., Ebola and Marburg] and arenaviruses [e.g., Lassa and Machupo])	Brucellosis (*Brucella* species) Epsilon toxin of *Clostridium perfringens* Food safety threats (e.g., *Salmonella* species, *Escherichia coli* O157:H7, and *Shigella*) Glanders (*Burkholderia mallei*) Melioidosis (*Burkholderia pseudomallei*) Psittacosis (*Chlamydia psittaci*) Q fever (*Coxiella burnetii*) Ricin toxin from *Ricinus communis* (castor beans) Staphylococcal enterotoxin B Typhus fever (*Rickettsia prowazekii*) Viral encephalitis (alphaviruses [e.g., Venezuelan equine encephalitis, eastern equine encephalitis, and western equine encephalitis]) Water safety threats (e.g., *Vibrio cholerae* and *Cryptosporidium parvum*)	Nipah virus Hantaviruses Tick-borne hemorrhagic fever viruses Tick-borne encephalitis viruses Yellow fever Multidrug-resistant tuberculosis

Rule 77: Sepsis is the final fatal biological syndrome

The early recognition and treatment of a septic patient irrespective of the presenting syndrome is essential for the reduction of mortality [1].

Sepsis is a Systemic Inflammatory Response Syndrome (SIRS) due to an infection. There are a number of causes of SIRS and some of these are shown in Figure 11.5.

The criteria for SIRS and thus sepsis are shown in Table 11.6. Early treatment of sepsis and specialist support is critical in order to prevent patient deterioration and the development of multi-organ failure (MOF). The presence of three or more systems failure is associated with over 50% mortality in the intensive therapy unit (ITU) population [2]. Management of sepsis includes the following [3]:

- Initial resuscitation
- Diagnosis
- Antibiotic therapy
- Source identification and control
- Fluid therapy
- Vasopressors
- Inotropic therapy
- Steroids
- Recombinant human-activated protein C
- Blood product administration

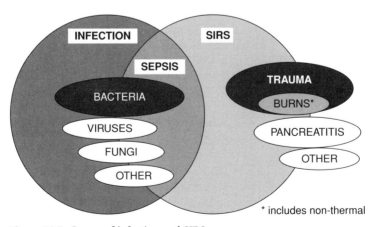

Figure 11.5 Causes of infection and SIRS.

Table 11.6 Criteria for sepsis and SIRS

Temperature	<36°C	>38.3°C
Heart rate	>90/min	
Systolic blood pressure	<90 mm Hg	
Respiratory rate	Tachypnoea	
White cell count (μL^{-1})	<4000	>12 000
Signs of organ dysfunction including hyperlactaemia, coagulopathy and altered conscious level		

- Mechanical ventilation strategies
- Sedation, analgesia and neuromuscular blockade
- Glucose control
- Renal replacement therapy
- Bicarbonate therapy
- Deep vein thrombosis prophylaxis
- Stress ulcer prophylaxis

References

1. Rivers E, Nguyen B, Havstad S, Ressler J, Muzzin A, Knoblich B, Peterson E, Tomlanovich M. Early goal-directed therapy in the treatment of severe sepsis and septic shock. *NEJM* 2001; **345**: 1368–1377.
2. Marshall JC, Cook DJ, Christou NV, Bernard GR, Sprung CL, Sibbald WJ. Multiple organ dysfunction score: a reliable descriptor of a complex clinical outcome. *Critical Care Medicine* 1995; **23**: 1638–1652.
3. Dellinger RP, Levy MM, Carlet JM, Bion J, Parker MM, Jaeschke R, Reinhart K, Angus DC, Brun-Buisson C, Beale R, Calandra T, Dhainaut JF, Gerlach H, Harvey M, Marini JJ, Marshall J, Ranieri M, Ramsay G, Sevransky J, Thompson BT, Townsend S, Vender JS, Zimmerman JL, Vincent JL. Surviving sepsis campaign: international guidelines for management of severe sepsis and septic shock. *Intensive Care Medicine* 2008; **34**: 17–60 and *Critical Care Medicine* 2008; **36**: 296–327.

Rule 78: Time–distance–shielding: the three principles of radiation protection

The most important feature of ionising radiation is that it is detectable with the right equipment. However, unlike most chemical hazards, radiation does not give an exposed person a feeling of being exposed. It is therefore necessary to identify and recognise radiation sources. Any radiation source should be identified with a trefoil warning symbol. Under the United Nations classification, radiation hazards are a designated Class 7 hazard. Packaging also gives indication of the radioactivity of the source and likely dose rate, usually in Sv/hr at a certain distance.

Where there is a risk of encountering radiation sources, personnel may be issued dosimeters. Electronic Personal Dosimeters (EPDs) can realistically be issued to emergency services personnel. These devices typically have the capability to detect gamma or x-ray or beta radiation. Settings often include cumulative dose and dose rate alarm. Contamination monitors are also available and issued to all UK Emergency Department and Ambulance Services.

Any exposure to ionising radiation may result in adverse health effects. It is for this reason that exposures should be kept to 'As Low As Reasonably Practicable' (ALARP). In order to achieve this, especially where the hazard cannot be removed immediately, there are some principles of radiation protection. These principles are:

- Time
- Distance
- Shielding

Time

The absorbed dose is proportional to the length of time a person is exposed to a radiation source (dose = dose rate × time). By reducing the duration by a half, the total absorbed dose will be reduced by a half.

Distance

A radiation dose rate decreases with distance and obeys the inverse square rule. This means that by doubling the distance, the dose rate will be reduced by a factor of 4. So, if a person is 10 m from a source and the dose rate is 100 mSv/h, if that person then moves to be 20 m away, the radiation is reduced to a dose rate 25 mSv/h.

Shielding

Each type of ionising radiation has different physical properties. This means that some forms, such as alpha and beta radiation which are charged particles, interact more readily with matter; conversely, electromagnetic radiation, such as gamma and x-rays, has no mass and is more penetrating. In order to reduce the distance gamma and x-ray radiation can penetrate, shielding is required. Dose rate is therefore inversely proportional to the amount of shielding; doubling the shielding halves the dose rate.

Rule 79: The radiation may kill in years, but the trauma kills in minutes

Ionising radiation can cause damage to DNA within human tissue, which may lead to mutations and cancers. At very high levels (thousand times the average annual background radiation dose, or 150 000 chest x-rays), the damage will be significant enough to cause cell death and acute radiation syndrome (ARS). However, the levels of radiation required to cause ARS are difficult to generate unless there is a nuclear incident, or exposure for long enough to a highly potent radiation source. These sources are strictly regulated and are detectable.

A radiation dispersal device (RDD) or 'dirty bomb' if detonated will explode and spread radiation over an area. Those casualties close enough to have a significant radiation dose will be so close to the explosion to have a higher risk of death from the blast. Casualties further away from the seat of the explosion may have life-threatening injuries, such as catastrophic haemorrhage or tension pneumothorax, and be additionally contaminated.

In the latter case, the management of the trauma should take precedence as the traumatic injuries may kill in minutes while the radiation may cause a higher risk of cancer that may be fatal in a number of years time. Even in cases of high radiation doses, the ARS does not cause life-threatening complication for a number of days. For this reason, casualties with combined injuries (trauma and radiation) may need to be operated on first and triaged as such.

CHAPTER 12
The Last Rule

> ! Rule 80:   Publish or others may perish

Rule 80: Publish or others may perish

Many aspects of medicine have a robust scientific foundation and are supported by randomised controlled clinical trials. Disaster medicine is inherently disadvantaged.

The unpredictable time and nature of events makes planned prospective scientific evaluation difficult. This situation is compounded by both the location of many natural disasters (in countries with a poor health and research infrastructure) and the ethical challenge of undertaking randomised studies during such a crisis.

Much can still be learned from retrospectively evaluating system performance through compliance with guidelines (e.g. triage algorithms), audit of unexpected patient outcomes, and debriefing of staff. Sharing of experiences through peer-reviewed publication assists others to identify recurrent themes in system weakness and failure, with the opportunity to revise plans, and to integrate lessons into training programmes.

Education in very simple terms (and the context of disaster medicine) is learning from others' mistakes and successes; *experience* is learning from your own. Most clinicians in developed countries will never experience having to manage patients in a resource-poor environment with damaged infrastructure. Yet, this is not an excuse for lack of education – and those few who have the experience are encouraged to share it through publication.

Index